FOOD
LOVE
FAMILY

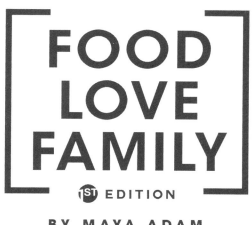

FOOD LOVE FAMILY

1ST EDITION

BY MAYA ADAM

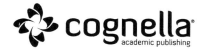

cognella®
academic publishing

Bassim Hamadeh, CEO and Publisher
Michael Simpson, Vice President of Acquisitions and Sales
Jamie Giganti, Senior Managing Editor
Miguel Macias, Graphic Designer
Kristina Stolte, Senior Field Acquisitions Editor
Michelle Piehl, Project Editor
Alexa Lucido, Licensing Coordinator

First published in the United States of America in 2016 by Cognella, Inc.

Cover photo taken by William Bottini.

Printed in the United States of America

ISBN: 978-1-63189-370-4 (pbk) / 978-1-63189-371-1 (br)

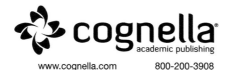

www.cognella.com   800-200-3908

DEDICATION

This book is dedicated to my parents

HERIBERT ADAM AND KOGILA MOODLEY

who inspired in me a love of cooking and a passion for teaching.

All author royalties will be donated to registered nonprofit organizations, including Just Cook for Kids, that support health and nutrition education for all.

CONTENTS

ACKNOWLEDGEMENTS

BY MAYA ADAM

This book would not have been published without the help of some extraordinary people. I would like to thank Hannah Kohrman, program manager at Just Cook for Kids and MD candidate 2019, for her wonderful contribution on sustainable eating and her support in making this book come alive. Thank you also to our contributing authors, Karen LeBillon, Jenny Rosenstrach, Jessica Almy, and Laura O'Donohue for their expertise and their generous contributions to this work. To Jamie Oliver and his team, we are honored to have your support. Karen Della Corte spent many hours during the summer of 2014 researching food allergies in children and prenatal nutrition for me as she prepared to welcome her own baby into the world. My editor, Michelle Piehl, and her team at Cognella have been a pleasure to work with. Here at the Stanford School of Medicine, my perspectives on nutrition have been shaped by conversations with Christopher Gardner and the writings of Berkeley's incomparably sensible Michael Pollan. All the while, Tim Dang, who has been both a student and a collaborator, has fearlessly attempted to sharpen my knife skills!

On the other side of the balance, I would like to thank my wonderful family. Lawrence, my husband and best friend, has patiently taken part in almost daily conversations about nutrition, health, and education—even though his professional passions lie elsewhere. My sister Kanya has been a constant reminder of the fact that healthy family meals can be thrown together by busy parents with celebratory ease and impressive flair. Mama, thank you for teaching me how to cook and for the many hours you spent cooking for us after you, yourself, returned home from a full-time teaching job at the university. Papa, thank you for teaching me to find joy in persevering until the job is done. Finally, I want to thank three people who are the inspiration for this book: Kiran, Misha and Milan, my beautiful boys, I have loved every minute we've spent together inside the kitchen and out of it! You continue to amaze me with your kindness, your joyfulness, and your beautiful personalities. Each and every day, you remind me to celebrate life.

Many thanks to you all…

— **Maya**

FOREWORD
BY JAMIE OLIVER

Encouraging everyone to cook from scratch and share and enjoy that food with their loved ones has always been at the heart of what I do. This book provides parents and caregivers around the world with knowledge and practical advice that will enable them to feed their children using good sense and a do-it-yourself mindset. From baby's first meal to the flavour adventures of older childhood, as parents we have the power to shape our children's food preferences. By teaching them to enjoy real food, made simply with love, we can set them up for a lifetime of good health and happiness.

— Jamie Oliver

To read more about Jamie Oliver's ongoing efforts to educate children about food and inspire families to cook, visit the Jamie Oliver Food Foundation at

http://www.jamieoliverfoodfoundation.org

CHAPTER 1

CHILD NUTRITION AND SOCIETY

The food our children eat has an enormous impact on their health and development. From the moment they're born, children are involved in an extreme sport called growth. Infants will spend as much as 38% of the energy they take in just to sustain their growth.[1] The ability to fight off disease, heal from injuries, and achieve developmental milestones like walking, talking, and learning at school are all dependent on a steady input of the right fuel: good nutrition.

Besides fueling growth and development, food plays many other important roles in our children's lives. Meals are a way for families to connect and a safe forum in which children can learn the skills of communication, share their concerns, and gain valuable social skills. Through food, traditions are passed from one generation to the next and children learn about where they come from, who they are and, in some ways, who they want to be.

Of course, not all kinds of food support our children's healthy growth and development equally. While children certainly need energy in the form of calories, where those calories come from is important too. Growing bodies need the right balance of specialized building blocks as well as the energy to build. When building a house, the quality of the raw materials matters. The same can be said for the raw materials (food) that contribute to the growth and development of a child. To take that analogy a few steps further, when a contractor is building a house, she knows that the foundations have to be solid, or the

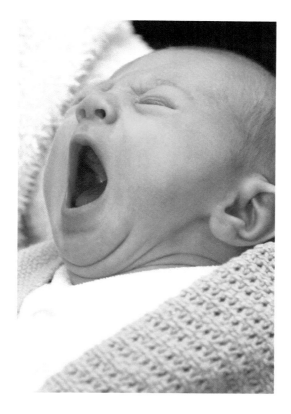

Figure 1.1   Infants use up to 38% of their energy intake to fuel growth.

house will be unstable and less likely to withstand stresses. The house needs to be held together by small but critical components like good-quality screws and strong nails. We can think of these as the vitamins and minerals that are critically important for our children's health, even though they're only needed in relatively small amounts. Finally, in order to make a house a home, it needs to be filled with love. Our children's food should be made with love too. When we outsource the job of feeding our children, by choosing too many highly processed foods, for example, we sacrifice the quality of the raw materials that are available to support their health. In general, processed food manufacturers have a major, vested interest in generating profits and comparatively little interest in protecting the long-term health of the people who consume their food. The opposite is true when a parent or loving caregiver cooks a family meal using mostly whole food ingredients.

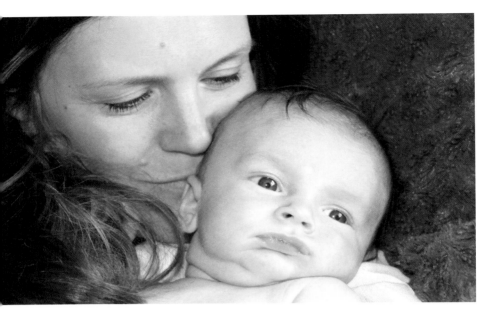

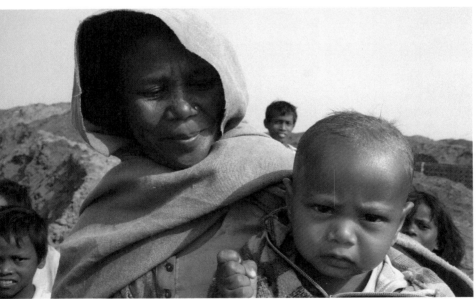

Figure 1.2.1-1.2.4 Feeding choices are influenced by the culture into which a child is born.

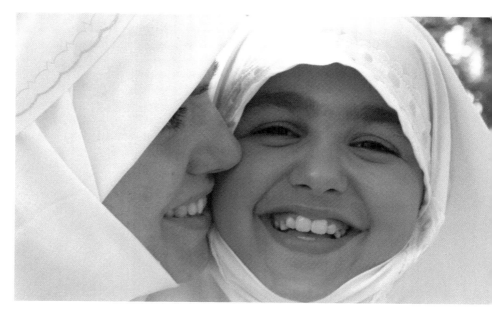

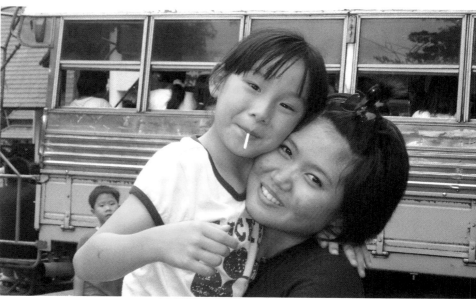

Families around the world have very different ways of feeding their children and many of these choices are influenced by the culture into which a child is born. The questions of what, when, how, and how much to eat are largely defined by what's considered normal or desirable within the family, the neighborhood, and even the country that a child calls home.

The environment in which children grow up significantly affects the foods they end up eating and, in this way, the environment will affect their long-term health. We see examples of this when we look at the very different collections of nutritional problems faced by children growing up in developed and developing countries.

In developed countries, like the United States, children are much more likely to be overfed, and have diets that are too high in nutrient-poor, calorie-dense foods. Diets like this, that are chronically low in nutrient density, raise a child's risk of suffering from over-nutrition, a form of malnutrition that often leads to chronic conditions of excess, like overweight and obesity in childhood. Childhood obesity raises the risk of many other chronic diseases, like heart disease and diabetes. The culture of eating in many developed countries, like the US, has developed to favor a model in which the consumption of excessive amounts of low-quality nutrition is all too often the norm. This trend is fueled by economic factors that make low-cost, highly processed foods readily available to families in these parts of the world.

In contrast, if we look at the developing world, children growing up in resource-poor areas may be more likely to suffer from under-nutrition due to insufficient availability of adequate foods. These children may end up deficient in protein or total calories and the under-nutrition that results comes with a separate list of health risks and complications. Under-nourished children often suffer from immune suppression, meaning that their bodies cannot effectively fight off infectious diseases.

What other factors influence the foods our children end up eating? At the level of the family, there are many factors that influence food choices: What resources (including time and money) does the family have to devote to buying and preparing fresh, healthful food? In parts of the world where access to electricity and running water are limited, safe food preparation as well as access to ingredients can be a major stumbling block for parents who may find themselves unable to provide nutritious meals for their growing children. The number of children in any given family also affects the distribution of resources. So, in parts of the world where women may not have access to contraception, large numbers of children may place an economic burden on

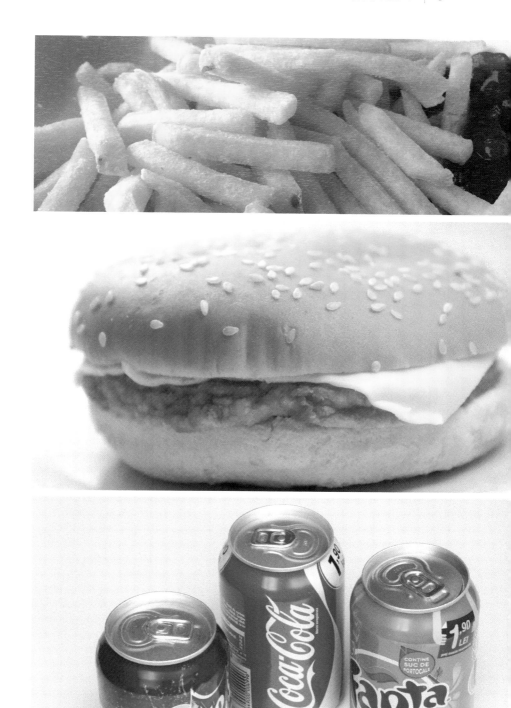

Figure 1.3. In many developed countries, the overconsumption of processed food has led to high rates of childhood obesity.

families, negatively affecting the nutrition status of children. In the United States and other developed parts of the world, parents may feel they don't have time to prepare healthful meals for their children or they may feel they lack the skills necessary to cook a balanced meal. Perhaps these barriers seem trivial at first, especially when compared with the profound lack of resources seen in other parts of the world. But, whenever parents and caregivers find themselves unable to provide nutritious foods for their children on a regular basis, the long-term health of those children will suffer.

The education available to parents and caregivers also plays a large role in defining the nutritional status of our children. When parents are educated about the importance of good nutrition, they are often more likely to subtly reallocate resources, no matter how limited those resources may be, in support of their children. Parents who have received even a basic exposure to nutrition education will be better equipped to prepare balanced meals and make healthier decisions about how, when, where, and how much to eat.

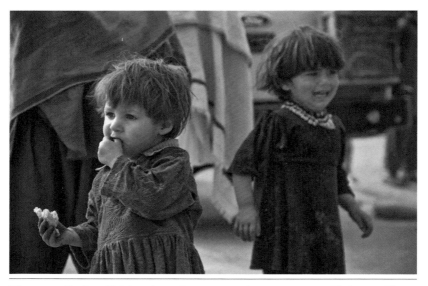

Figure 1.4   Children in under-resourced areas are more likely to suffer from under-nutrition.

Does the family eat together on a regular basis? Studies have shown many health and other benefits of eating regular family meals.[2] These benefits aren't limited to better nutritional intake, but also encompass psychosocial benefits that can set a child up for success in multiple arenas.

If we consider the neighborhood in which a child is growing up, we encounter other questions: Are fresh, whole foods readily available at a local supermarket or are convenience stores the predominant source of food? What foods are served at school? Is there a weekly farmers' market anywhere in the vicinity? Access to fresh, real food ingredients is still tragically limited for many families around the world. Yet, this reality shouldn't make us throw up our hands in despair and give up on the idea that healthy, home-cooked meals can save our children's lives. We need to focus as much energy on eradicating food deserts as we do on educating families about how they can take their health into their own hands by cooking simple, healthful meals. When the culture of eating at home is one that promotes health, a long-term investment is made in the future of the children growing up there.

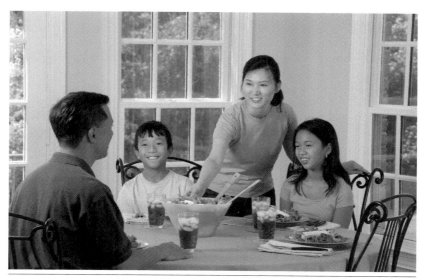

Figure 1.5 Studies have shown significant health benefits associated with eating regular family meals.

Even on the national level, the culture of eating influences the foods offered to a child living in any given country. For example, in France, children snack infrequently when compared with children growing up in America. In France, the culture of eating discourages frequent snacking, as the French believe that frequent snacking can lead to dysregulation of healthy cycles of hunger and eating. In the US, in contrast, frequent snacking is sometimes believed to modulate behavior in young children and parents are advised to have snacks on hand in order to avoid letting children get hungry, as this is believed to lead to temper tantrums and other behavioral aberrations. Even at the level of government, legislature like farm subsidies for certain agricultural products and food marketing regulations have an influence on what a child in any given country ends up eating. Here in the US, the government has historically incentivized farmers to grow large amount of things like corn and soy. This had led to an overabundance of these agricultural products and, as a consequence, they have become cheap and available substrates for processed food manufacturers to use in a large variety of processed food products. Compared with many countries in Europe, processed food manufacturers in the US are given considerable freedom to choose how the products they manufacture are marketed, even when they are being marketed to children.

From the macroscopic level of government regulations to the microscopic level of the child and her immediate family, all of these environmental factors play a part in determining the foods a child eats. In this way, the environment contributes to the overall health outcomes of children around the world.

Most parents around the world share the desire to protect their offspring from acute and chronic health problems. Childhood is a sensitive period for healthy growth and bonding between children and their caregivers. Food can be an important part of both of those critical childhood experiences. By teaching our children to enjoy reasonable amounts of healthy food, ideally prepared by a loving parent or caregiver, we can set them up for a lifetime of good health and happiness. Food is much more than just fuel for our children's growing bodies. Perhaps one of the most valuable gifts that we can give to our children is the gift of feeding them—and ourselves—mindfully and with love.

CHAPTER 2

WELCOME TO THE MILKY WAY: INTRODUCTION TO INFANT FEEDING

From the moment our children are delivered into our arms, we take on the responsibility of providing them with food. This responsibility can be both exhilarating and terrifying, especially for first-time parents. The biggest challenge: newborn babies don't come with personalized feeding instructions! No matter how many educational materials new parents have read, the day they need to start making decisions about when, where, how, and how much to feed their own newborns is often a day of great excitement as well as great anxiety.

One of the earliest choices made by women all over the world on the day they become mothers is whether to feed their babies breast milk or infant formula. For many parents, this decision is not as simple as it may seem and involves a careful assessment of the risks and benefits of each of these feeding methods. The factors that affect the choice between breast milk and formula differ greatly around the world and they're rooted in the diverse fields of physiology, history, culture, and economics, as we'll see later on in this chapter. The majority of medical experts and health regulatory bodies around the world recognize that, for most babies, breast milk provides the best and most complete form of nutrition for the first six months of life[1] and that supplemental breastfeeding should be continued until the child is at least one year of age. However, the challenges faced by new mothers are significant enough that global rates of exclusive breastfeeding remain significantly lower than the targets set by heath protection agencies like the World Health Organization[2]. Let's explore infant feeding to try to better understand the many factors involved in the question: What should I feed my baby?

THE HUMAN BREAST: AN ON-DEMAND MILK-MAKING MACHINE

The human breast in an amazing organ, specially designed for feeding human offspring. In both men and women, the breast contains mammary glands, but in females, these glands are programmed to respond to sex hormones like estrogen around the time of puberty. Exposure to these sex hormones leads to breast development.

The main function of the mammary glands is to make, briefly store, and secrete breast milk to feed the human infant. Breast milk drains to the nipple via lactiferous ducts, where each duct has its own small opening. Surrounding the nipple, a darker area of skin, called the areola, helps the human infant locate the source of food. When babies are born, their eyesight is still developing, but they can make out light and dark objects. This is where the areola is helpful in locating the nipple. The remainder of the breast is composed of connective tissue (collagen and elastin) and adipose tissue, or fat. The entire breast is supported and anchored to the chest wall by Cooper's ligaments.

Milk production follows a supply-and-demand rhythm: as the baby grows and the demand for milk increases, more milk is produced. Because of this, the first weeks of breastfeeding are very important in establishing an adequate supply of breast milk. If the breast is not stimulated by early infant suckling, the mammary glands respond by shutting down milk production. Even if the stimulus for milk production is insufficient (for example, when babies are combination-fed with infant formula from birth), it will likely be more difficult for the mammary glands to catch up and the amount of milk produced may be insufficient for exclusive breastfeeding. In cases where babies and their mothers are physically separated in the early weeks of life, due to maternal birth complications or other extenuating circumstances, a breast pump can be used to mimic the early stimulus for milk production, preserving the mother's ability to produce breast milk. This means that babies who are born prematurely can receive breast milk, even if they are initially unable to successfully latch on and feed directly from the breast.

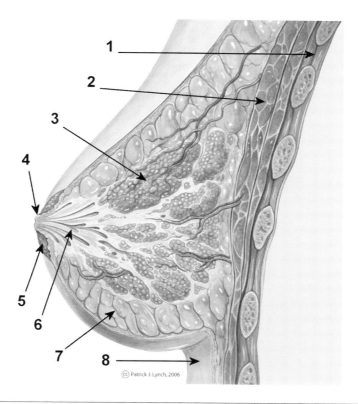

Figure 2.1   Anatomy of the Human Breast. The first few weeks of breastfeeding can be a challenging period as mother and baby learn a new skill.

1. *Cooper's ligaments anchor the breast to the chest wall*
2. *Connective tissue (collagen and elastin) support and anchor the breast*
3. *Mammary glands synthesize and secrete breast milk*
4. *The nipple is the part of the breast where milk is ejected*
5. *The darkened areola helps baby locate the nipple*
6. *Lactiferous ducts drain milk from the mammary glands to the areola*
7. *Adipose tissue cushions, protects, and supports mammary glands*
8. *Chest wall provides stability to the breast*

SYNCHRONIZED REFLEXES: HOW BREASTFEEDING WORKS

Healthy newborn babies come equipped with a host of impressive reflexes that help them take in enough food to survive. The rooting reflex, for example, causes a newborn infant to turn her head toward anything that strokes her cheek or mouth. She'll then open her mouth and move her head around until the object that touched her cheek (ideally, it's her mother's nipple) is located. This reflex is present from birth in the healthy infant, as is the ability to suck and swallow—an impressive feat of coordination for someone so small. When a baby gets hungry and begins to feed at the breast, a chain of events occurs that make up another highly coordinated reflex involving both mother and child: the let-down reflex. The infant's suckling sends sensory information to a part of the mother's brain called the hypothalamus. When the hypothalamus receives this information, it begins to modulate the release of hormones in order to facilitate the delivery of milk. Firstly, the hypothalamus triggers the release of a hormone called oxytocin from the posterior part of the mother's pituitary gland, another part of the brain. This hormone causes the contraction of small muscle cells lining the mammary glands in which breast milk is stored. The contraction of these cells causes milk to be ejected through the lactiferous ducts and out into the infant's mouth. At the same time, the hypothalamus sends another signal to the anterior part of the mother's pituitary gland that causes the release of a hormone called prolactin. Prolactin acts on the mammary glands to stimulate the production of more milk. In this way, milk can be ready for consumption whenever the baby is hungry and, just as she starts feeding, the process of producing new milk is already underway.

Interestingly, the mechanical stimulus of the infant suckling at the breast isn't the only way in which this reflex is triggered. Just the sound of an infant's cry can result in this cascade of hormone release and milk ejection from the breast. Crying is actually considered a relatively late indicator of hunger in babies. They will first root around trying to locate their food source somewhere nearby. Only when the situation starts to become more urgent will newborns cry for their food. This makes a lot of sense, as that cry will likely draw the attention of their caregiver and, as we now know, start the process of releasing and making milk for the next meal.

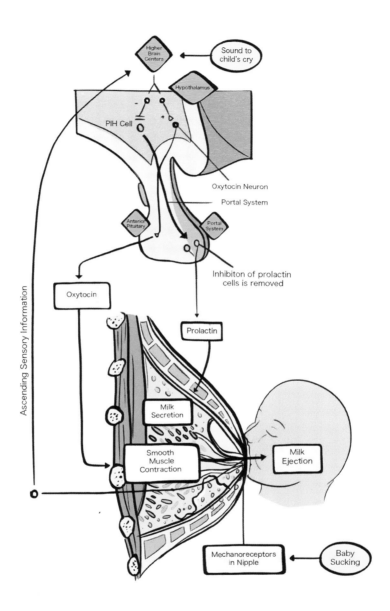

Figure 2.2   The Let-Down Reflex
Illustrated by Lavanya Mahadevan

Lila is a 30-year-old first-time mother of a healthy newborn boy. Both she and her husband Xavier have been counting down the days until the birth of this child and the new parents have certainly done their homework! They've read all about the benefits of breastfeeding, purchased a special feeding pillow (which Lila brought with her to the hospital when she went into labor), and are committed to following the recommendations of pediatric health authorities. They plan to breastfeed baby Jake exclusively until six months of age and continue with supplemental breast-feeding until at least a year of age.

Lila works as a teacher at the local high school and is eager to return to work for the start of the new school year, which falls around six weeks after her estimated delivery date. At the school, there is a dedicated feeding room for breastfeeding mothers on the staff; Xavier, who has flexible working hours, will be able to bring the baby to school for regular feedings. Lila has even drafted a tentative four-hour feeding schedule for the early months, which she hopes to implement by gently establishing a routine in which her baby feeds at 8:00 a.m., 12:00 p.m., 4:00 p.m., and so on.

The delivery goes smoothly and Lila is told that she has a healthy newborn, weighing 7.5 lbs (just over 3.4 kg). Soon after the delivery, the maternity nurse suggests that Lila try breastfeeding Jake. The nurse helps Lila to find a comfortable position and, after several tries, baby Jake is able to latch briefly on one side. Lila is somewhat concerned because she's unsure whether her baby actually received any milk during his first feed and she suspects her milk hasn't even come in yet, as she doesn't yet feel the breast fullness described in the book she read on success-ful lactation. The nurse reassures her that successful breastfeeding usually takes practice—both for her and the newborn—and Lila is advised to rest for a few hours before trying again.

For the rest of the afternoon, Jake appears to be hungry every couple of hours and Lila tries feeding him, with the support of the maternity nurse. She's surprised by the fact that the feeding is actually a bit uncomfortable and the nurse tries to help baby Jake take more of the areola into his mouth, thereby relieving some of the tension on the tender skin of the nipples. Jake appears to be getting quite hungry now and Lila feels that his cries are sounding more desperate. That night, Lila feels changes in her breasts that signal her that she's now producing milk and the feeding cycles continue through the night. Jake is slowly getting better at latching, but Lila is exhausted and her nipples are raw and bleeding slightly. Every time Jake feeds, Lila has to brace herself for the pain of the initial latch, but again the nurse reassures her that this is normal in the early days of breastfeeding. By day three, Lila realizes that her planned four-hourly feeding schedule is going to be harder

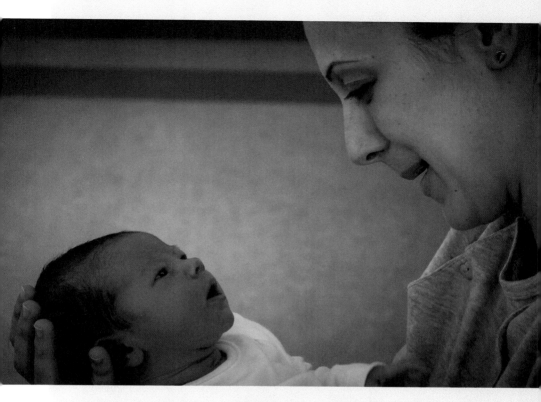

Figure 2.3   The first few weeks of breastfeeding can be a challenging period as mother and baby learn a new skill. Support from health care providers and family is very important as breast-feeding is established.

to accomplish than she had anticipated. She is exhausted and teary and worried about her baby, who has lost 5% of his birth weight. Now, back at home, Lila sends Xavier to the pharmacy to buy some infant formula. She feels deeply disappointed that her experience of breastfeeding wasn't what she had expected and, desperate for sleep, she feeds the baby a small amount of infant formula after which both mother and baby sleep for five hours—the longest period of sleep Lila's had since Jake was born.

Lila awakens to the sound of her baby's cry and Xavier asks her if she'd like to try breastfeeding again now that she's had some rest. The new mother is hesitant and the couple discusses the option of giving up on breastfeeding altogether, but Xavier encourages her to try for just one more day. The new mother agrees and day four of breastfeeding feels easier and much less painful. Lila is encouraged by the fact that her baby now seems to be getting more breast milk from her with each feed and he's sleeping longer between feeds. When the maternity nurse does a home-visit the following day, she advises Lila to discontinue the supplemental formula feeding now that breastfeeding is going well.

After several weeks, both Lila and Jake are completely comfortable with breast-feeding and the baby is gaining weight appropriately and thriving. Lila still hasn't managed to maintain a regular feeding schedule, so she decides to rent a breast pump, enabling her to return to work as planned, while Xavier takes over some of the daily feeding responsibilities. At work, the staff lactation room provides Lila with a place to pump and store her breast milk in a refrigerator. By the time Jake is six months of age, Jake and Lila are happy, healthy, and ready to embark on the adventures of solid foods, in addition to breastfeeding. By the time Jake is one year of age, Lila and Jake both still enjoy their special shared bonding time during breastfeeds, so Lila continues supplemental breastfeeding until Jake is two years old. Looking back, Lila feels happy that she decided to persevere during the challenging early days of breastfeeding. She also feels grateful for the encouragement she received from those around her.

WHY BREAST IS (USUALLY) BEST: THE BENEFITS OF BREASTFEEDING

Next we're going to look at some of the benefits of breastfeeding for the infant, the mother, and the community. One thing to keep in mind as you read these benefits is that there are some mothers who, for health or logistical reasons, are unable to breastfeed their babies. For these women, reading about the benefits of breastfeeding can be anxiety-provoking and they can come away feeling that they have already failed as parents because they are not able to provide these benefits to their child. Like all decisions on infant care, the choice of infant feeding method should be made after careful consideration of the risks and benefits of each alternative. While breastfeeding offers the advantages discussed below, many loving parents have raised perfectly healthy children with the help of infant formula. Safe formula feeding, in parts of the world where water supplies are reliable and resources for safe bottle-feeding are available, can certainly end up being a sensible choice for some families. For most healthy babies and mothers, however, the benefits of breastfeeding usually outweigh the risks. Let's review some of these benefits in the sections below:

BENEFITS OF BREASTFEEDING FOR THE INFANT

Human milk is species-specific and actually changes in composition as the baby grows. The first milk, called colostrum, is a thick, yellowish fluid that's rich in protein and antibodies, also called immunoglobulins. The antibodies in colostrum protect the newborn from an enormous number of unfamiliar microbes in the environment. Coming from the sterile environment of the mother's uterus, the newborn is bombarded with potential pathogens. The mother's body has been working hard to develop antibodies that can protect her and her baby from the specific microbes in their shared environment. Because these tailor-made antibodies can pass from mother to child through breast milk, passive immunity is one of the major benefits of breastfeeding and can be lifesaving during disease outbreaks or in places where water supplies are contaminated. Colostrum gradually changes into mature breast milk by day three or four of the newborn's life. Mature breast milk is higher in sugar and fat than colostrum, but it also contains appropriate amounts of all the nutrients necessary to support growth, including protein and water. For the duration of breastfeeding, antibodies from the mother are passed via breast milk to the infant. This is one of the main reasons young children experience frequent illnesses after being weaned from the breast.

In addition to providing protection from infectious diseases, breastfeeding has been shown to reduce a child's risk of developing diabetes and asthma and some studies have even linked breastfeeding to a lower risk of obesity and sudden infant death syndrome (SIDS).

Finally, several studies done over the past decade have suggested a connection between breastfeeding and higher IQ scores later in life, but it remains unclear whether the relationship is a causal one. A 2007 review of the literature conducted by the World Health Organization suggested that breastfeeding was associated with increased cognitive development in children but that it remained unclear whether the association was due to compounds found in breast milk or whether the enhanced bonding between mother and child that can occur during breastfeeding contributes to the intellectual development of the child. An intense debate continues over whether or not the findings of increased IQ in breastfed children is in fact directly related to the breast milk.[3]

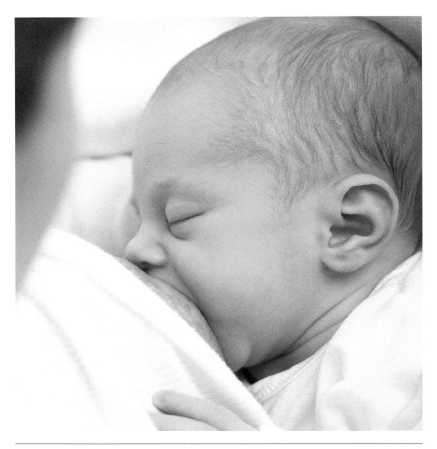

Figure 2.4   Human breastmilk provides species-specific, tailored nutrition and protection from infections, among other benefits.

BENEFITS OF BREASTFEEDING FOR THE MOTHER

For mothers, particularly in the developing world, there are some significant advantages to breastfeeding. The first, and perhaps most obvious of these, is that breastfeeding is a cost-effective way of feeding a child. In parts of the world where resources are scarce, the cost of formula feeding can be crippling for many families, while breastfeeding is associated with a comparatively small cost to the mother.

Frequent breastfeeding also delays the return of the menstrual cycle and can be an effective way of supporting adequate birth-spacing, especially in parts of the world where women lack easy access to contraceptives. In parts of the world where women may not have access to contraception for cultural or economic reasons, multiple births in rapid succession can place an enormous burden on the family. This burden is partly an economic one because more mouths to feed means more financial pressure on the family. However, multiple successive pregnancies also take a major toll on the health of the mother and, in so doing, it negatively affects the wellbeing of the family.

There is also a growing body of evidence suggesting that early skin-to-skin contact between mother and child leads to more successful bonding and improved overall health for both mother and child. These findings have led to recommendations that healthy newborns should be placed in skin-to-skin contact with their mothers almost immediately after birth. This practice, also called "kangaroo care," has the added benefit of preventing hypothermia in the newborn and is thought to facilitate successful breastfeeding. One of the effects of the hormones involved in the let-down reflex (prolactin and oxytocin) is that they can relax the mother and make her more inclined to nurture her baby. Oxytocin also helps the uterus to contract to its original size and this reduces the risk of postpartum bleeding.

For women who breastfeed for eight months or more, the long-term health benefits include reduced risk of developing breast cancer, ovarian cancer, and osteoporosis.[4]

BENEFITS OF BREASTFEEDING FOR THE COMMUNITY

There are also some benefits to the community and environment that make breastfeeding a good choice for mothers who decide on this method of infant feeding. Compared with formula feeding, breastfeeding produces relatively little waste. There are no cans, bottles, silicon nipples, labels, or packaging associated with breastfeeding. Breastfeeding also reduces healthcare costs associated with the higher rates of infections and hospitalizations seen in formula-fed babies. These are some of the added benefits to society when mothers choose to breastfeed.

WHAT HAPPENED TO BREASTFEEDING? A BRIEF HISTORY OF INFANT FEEDING

With so many health benefits associated with the act of breastfeeding, it may be surprising to see that global rates of exclusive breastfeeding in infants under six months of age, in both developed and developing countries, remain low, ranging from 20% in central and eastern European countries to 44% in South Asia.[2]

What happened to breastfeeding around the world? The answer to this question is deeply rooted in the cultural shifts in infant feeding that have occurred around the world over the past five or six decades. Those shifts were motivated by some specific health challenges in the early part of the twentieth century, by the innovations that were developed to try to address those challenges, and by the exploitation of those innovations for the financial gain of large corporations. In the early 1900s infant mortality rates in many parts of the world, including the US, were relatively high. Many of these deaths were thought to be the result of substandard or improper infant feeding. In the US, this gave rise to two new professions: pediatrics and food science. Food scientists began studying questions about food quality—whether pasteurized was better than raw cow's milk and what could be added to it to make it more nutritious. At the same time, in Europe, scientists were also searching for a nutritious substitute for breast milk designed specifically for infants whose mothers were unable to breastfeed or had died in childbirth (another health outcome that occurred more frequently in the early 1900s.) When scientists in Europe invented the first commercial infant formulas, Americans were ready to welcome this long-sought-after innovation. A new medical specialty, pediatrics, came into being and one of the primary tasks of early pediatricians was to prescribe infant formula in increasing doses to support the healthy growth of infants who lacked access to breast milk. Initially, infant formula could be used only under the careful guidance of a physician. It didn't take long for the manufacturers of infant formula to see the potential for making a sizable profit out of their discovery. Formula manufacturers began aggressively marketing their product as not just an *acceptable* substitute for breast milk, but also a *superior* form of infant feeding. Advertisements showing healthy babies who had ostensibly been raised on formula were used widely to increase the sales and popularity of breast-milk substitutes. As the demand for these formulas grew, they became available to the general public without a prescription—just as we can walk into a pharmacy and buy a can of infant formula today. Within a decade, mothers and medical professionals alike began to believe that formula was not only a safe alternative to breastfeeding, but also a superior one. By the early 1970s approximately three quarters of American infants were fed exclusively with commercial infant formulas.

By this time, however, birth rates in industrialized parts of the world were declining, so the formula manufacturers went in search of new markets. Advertising campaigns were launched in many developing countries, but because resources, including clean water, were scarce in many of those regions, mortality rates among infants who were bottle fed with commercial formula increased sharply.[5]

THE IMPORTANCE OF BREASTFEEDING IN PLACES WHERE RESOURCES ARE SCARCE

There are two effects of breastfeeding that, while beneficial in the developed world, are frequently lifesaving when we look at the developing world. In the developing world, where water supplies are not always clean and where the resources for proper sterilization of bottles are often not available, the formula itself becomes a major source of infectious disease in babies. Children under the age of five, especially young infants, can rapidly become dehydrated when they succumb to diarrheal diseases (caused by infections of the gut). Especially in developing parts of the world, where sanitation may be inadequate, diarrheal disease is a common cause of infant mortality.[6] To make matters worse, when contaminated formula is given to a child who is not receiving the passive immunity from her mother's breast milk, the risk of developing an infection is increased. Finally, the economics of formula feeding in the developing world also plays a part in the high number of deaths seen in under-resourced parts of the world. When parents spend a large portion of their weekly income on relatively expensive infant formulas, the necessity to use the formula sparingly increases significantly. This means that many mothers will try to stretch the formula by diluting it, leading to the potential for malnutrition of the child. When a child is malnourished, her immune system becomes less capable of protecting her from infectious agents—like the microbes found in formula prepared with contaminated water. Where water supplies are unsafe, infants who are bottle fed are significantly more likely to die from gastrointestinal infections than breastfed babies are.[7]

CASE STUDY 2.2

Nosizwe is a 22-year-old new mother living in the township of Khayelitsha, just outside of Cape Town, South Africa. She lives with her mother and older sister in a small shack near the highway that leads into town. The family collects their water from a communal tap a few minutes away and it's Nosizwe's job to carry a large plastic bucket of water, from the tap to their home, on her head every other day. The bucket is stored in the shack and water is used sparingly for washing and drinking, and cooking over a paraffin stove. Nosizwe worked at a fast food restaurant in the city until six months ago when she lost her job and, since then, she has helped at home by looking after her sister's child while waiting for her own baby to arrive. When Nosizwe's daughter finally arrives late one night, delivered by a community volunteer nurse at the small local clinic, the new mother is very happy to meet her beautiful little girl. Emilie weighs 6 lbs (2.72 kg) at birth and is found to be perfectly healthy. Nosizwe asks the volunteer nurse how she should feed the child and the nurse tells Nosizwe it this is her decision to make, but the clinic can give her free samples of formula if she decides to bottle feed the baby. Nosizwe looks at the posters taped to the clinic walls, showing pictures of healthy-looking, formula-fed babies, and she remembers that her own sister chose to bottle feed her child. She decides to accept the formula samples and even receives several coupons for store discounts on formula to use once the samples have run out.

For the first six weeks of her life, Emilie seems to be doing well. She feeds eagerly, appears to be gaining weight, and learns how to smile at the loving, familiar faces around her. When the formula samples have run out, Nosizwe

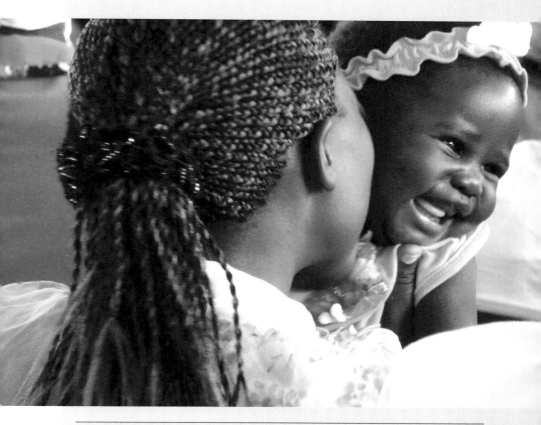

Figure 2.5 In parts of the world with limited access to clean water and the financial resources needed for safe formula feeding, exclusive breastfeeding saves many children's lives.

begins to use the coupons at the store, but she's surprised at how much the baby now drinks. The cans of powdered formula seem to run empty more quickly every week and she starts to worry that soon, she may not have enough money to pay for the food Emilie needs to continue growing. The combined household income is smaller now that Nosizwe is no longer working and there's little left over to pay for the expensive cans of formula. Trying to plan for the weeks ahead, Nosizwe gradually begins to dilute Emilie's formula—trying hard to make each can of powder last just a few days longer. At first the baby hardly seems to notice, but over the next few weeks, she becomes thinner and seems less interactive than she once was. One morning, when Nosizwe is changing her daughter, she notices that the baby has passed watery, greenish stools and over the next few days, the diarrhea continues. Emilie now begins to look emaciated and lethargic, so the worried mother takes her back to the local clinic. After a long walk in the heat, mother and daughter wait for several hours to see the single doctor who visits this clinic once a week to see a long line-up of patients. After examining Emilie, the doctor tells Nosizwe that her daughter is severely underweight for her age and that she has likely been infected with a pathogen in the water used to mix her formula. Nosizwe is told to feed her as frequently as possible for the next few days, mixing the formula exactly according to the instructions. The doctor gives Nosizwe three bags of infant formula powder and a special powder packet with mixing instructions to make an oral solution that will rehydrate the child. He tells Nosizwe that it's very important for her to boil and cool the water used for anything Emilie will be drinking and gives instructions on how to properly clean the baby's bottles. Emilie is to be brought back to the clinic in a week so that the doctor can weigh her and examine her again. Nosizwe follows the doctor's directions carefully and, luckily, Emilie recovers and begins gaining weight. At her follow-up visit, the doctor tells Nosizwe that Emilie is a very lucky girl. Without her mother's antibody-rich breast milk to protect her, she could easily have become fatally dehydrated from her diarrheal disease.

BREASTFEEDING AND HIV/AIDS

In many parts of the world where safe formula feeding is difficult to achieve, mother-to-child transmission of HIV is an accompanying concern. The virus can be transmitted through breast milk, but given the risks associated with unsafe formula feeding in these areas, exclusive breastfeeding is widely recommended as the safest alternative for most families. Simply put, the risk of dying due to diarrheal disease from unsafe bottle feeding is higher than the risk of contracting HIV via exclusive breastfeeding. The practice of combination feeding—alternating between breast milk and formula—is strongly discouraged in cases where the mother is HIV positive. The reason for this is that the gut lining of infants who ingest contaminated infant formula can become inflamed secondary to infection from the waterborne microbes. The inflamed gut wall is more porous, allowing any viral particles containing HIV to more easily gain access to the body of the child. Combination feeding significantly raises the risk of mother-to-child HIV transmission and carries an increased risk of causing diarrheal disease in the child. In short, for mothers living in places where safe formula feeding is not feasible, exclusive breastfeeding is usually the safest feeding practice. Antiretroviral treatment further reduces the risk of mother-to-child HIV transmission.[8]

SAFE FORMULA FEEDING

In parts of the world where formula feeding can be safely accomplished, mothers who choose this method of feeding also need to receive adequate support from their healthcare providers, family, and community during the trying postnatal period. Mothers who choose formula feeding should be advised to follow formula preparation instructions carefully, never diluting the mixture. It's imperative that clean water be used for this purpose and any water suspected of carrying contaminants be sterilized by allowing it to boil for several minutes before cooling it in a sterile container. Formula should be prepared shortly before feeding time and formula that's been kept at room temperature for longer periods of time should be discarded as pathogens grow quickly in warm, moist, nutrient-rich environments. Finally, mothers who are formula feeding, either by choice or by necessity, should be given good advice on how to maximize mother–child bonding during feeds; for example, by encouraging skin-to-skin bottle-feeding and kangaroo care (wearing the baby against the skin of the chest) for periods of the day when this is feasible for either parent. Ensuring adequate stress-free time for both parents to get to know their baby by simply being together is equally important.

The newborn period is often an emotionally trying one for new parents who are experiencing dramatic shifts in their roles and their lifestyle. New parents may suddenly find themselves with little control over their schedules as they adjust to the responsibilities of caring for another human being. This can also be a time of great anxiety about the health of the newborn, especially with regard to feeding, and feelings of inadequacy are common among new parents. Perhaps one of the most reassuring suggestions for new parents is that often, their parental instincts, grounded in common sense and based on an unconditional love for their child, will guide them in making the right decisions for the unique circumstances in which their family exists. There is no single "correct way" to feed or care for a new life. Approaching these tasks with a positive attitude, and ideally with plenty of support from the sidelines, will most likely lead to a favorable outcome.

Ultimately, happy parents—especially happy mothers—will have the best chance of making sensible feeding decisions and raising healthy babies. So, the support of the mother is a key factor in ensuring baby's nutrition and good health.

A NOTE ON VITAMIN D

Breast milk provides complete, ideal nutrition for human babies. However, exclusively breastfed babies in some parts of the world may require supplemental vitamin D on a daily basis. Vitamin D is a fat-soluble vitamin that facilitates the absorption of calcium and several other important nutrients. Together with calcium, vitamin D supports bone health and growth. We get vitamin D from two sources: it can be synthesized in the skin when the skin is exposed to sunlight. The second source of vitamin D is the food we eat. Breast milk is relatively low in vitamin D. For infants who live in parts of the world where their skin is exposed to little direct sunlight (because they're covered up with clothing, kept indoors most of the day, or living in a climate with little sunshine), daily vitamin D supplementation during exclusive breastfeeding is recommended.

Parent Forum

I have a confession to make: Sometimes, I feel like I'm living a dual life. In one, I'm a medical doctor who teaches classes on child health and nutrition. The rest of the time, I'm the mother of three young children trying (not always successfully) to make the right food choices for my family. Both of my personas live in a world where fast, highly processed foods are available on every street corner. The sheer number of food options is a recipe for confusion. And, like many parents, I often find myself struggling to make the right choices, against a tidal wave of food marketing messages that are screaming at me to just chill out and order pizza.

This is not a new feeling, this confusion over what to put in my children's mouths. It started ten years ago when a tiny, six-pound human being was delivered into my arms by a nurse who completely forgot to hand me the instruction manual. I had read a lot about the advantages of breastfeeding and I was convinced that I wanted to exclusively breast-feed my first child. But I was completely unprepared for the challenges associated with an activity that I had assumed would be a piece of cake. When the logistics of going back to medical school, three weeks postpar-tum, forced me to start supplementing my baby's diet with formula, I felt I had somehow already failed him as a mother. To add to my distress, I now had to choose which formula my precious newborn would drink (PS: they're all the same) and how he would drink it: glass or BPA-free plastic? Latex or silicone? Once again, the choices—and potential for making the wrong ones—seemed limitless. Despite those early struggles, I ended up enjoying the months and years I spent breastfeeding my children and there's no doubt in my mind that breast milk was the best nutritional choice for my babies. But as my children grew up, making the right food choices for them continued to feel a bit like navigating a minefield.

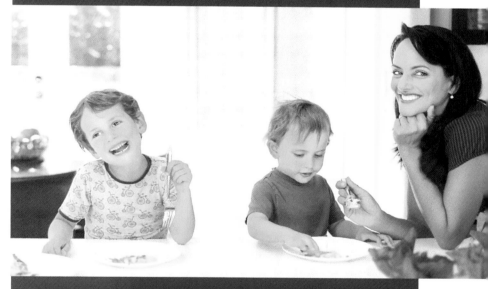

Figure 2.6   Adam and two of her three children. Her kitchen motto: "It's better to be real than to be perfect!"

It wasn't until my medical training landed me in a township nutrition clinic in South Africa that I realized the true origin of my maternal insecurities: I was spoiled. In fact, I was spoiled rotten by too many convenient options and too much time to second-guess my decisions. The mothers I met in South Africa didn't have these luxuries. Amid rampant HIV, poverty, malnutrition, domestic violence, and other crime, they were boldly raising children. It was almost unfathomable. I met a single mother, named Baselwa, who breastfed her twins in a one-room shack with no windows. The walls were made of laundry detergent boxes and her only source of water was the enormous bucket she carried on her head from a communal tap. (The twins were strapped tightly to her body with a large blanket while she walked.) Baselwa's determination to exclusively breastfeed her babies was based on the fact that she had seen too many formula-fed newborns die from diarrheal disease due to contaminated water and malnutrition. Without the antibody protection of their mother's milk, these babies simply couldn't fight off the pathogens that lurked in their formula bottles. Seeing Baselwa's limited options for feeding her babies, I suddenly felt embarrassed about the anxiety I had felt over my own feeding choices. Bottle or breast? Glass or plastic? Try life or death. Those were options I'd never really had to worry about.

In industrialized parts of the world, we often have so many choices, and so much time to contemplate those choices, that we end up doubting ourselves. Sometimes we even criticize the decisions of our peers to make ourselves feel better: "How could she stop breast feeding so soon?" or, later, "Can you believe she lets him eat that?" In contrast, I saw none of that judgment between the mothers I met in South Africa. Instead, they would listen to each other and trade feeding strategies. They would bring food and help cook a meal. They would look each other in the eye and say, "You are managing to care beautifully for this child." And they would *mean* it.

I don't wish for any of us to know, first hand, the struggles faced by the Baselwas of our world. But we can certainly learn a lot from these unsung heroes. As parents around the world try (from day one) to do the best they can with the resources available to them, perhaps the most important choice we can make is this: to feed our children with good sense, confidence, and love, supporting one another in the process.

CHAPTER 3
THE ADVENTURE OF A LIFETIME: INTRODUCING SOLIDS TO BABIES AROUND THE WORLD

INTRODUCING...FOOD!

Sometime around four to six months of age, healthy babies suddenly become interested in solid food. They begin to study adults and older children around them as these early role models engage in the act of eating and enjoying real food. In time, babies will start reaching for that food and they have a strong instinctive desire to put into their mouths everything they pick up. This "mouthing behavior" is believed to be important in the priming of the immune system, as babies are exposed to microbes in the world around them.[1] The propensity to put objects in the mouth may also be associated with teething[2] but the end result is that babies begin to learn even more about the world around them—and that world includes food. Using their mouths, babies begin to taste, feel, and otherwise explore the exciting new terrain of edible adventures.

For many first-time parents, beginning to feed their babies with solid foods can be a challenging task. New parents may feel unsure about their baby's developmental readiness for solids. They may also feel overwhelmed by the choice of which foods to introduce first and how to keep their baby safe from adverse food reactions or choking. For many parents, especially those who struggled to establish a regular, comfortable milk-feeding schedule in the early months, the prospect of having to learn yet another new set of skills can seem daunting. Introducing solids certainly does include a learning curve for everyone involved: Caregivers learn how to choose, prepare, and deliver solid foods while the recipients of that food learn how to navigate the intake of a new kind of nourishment. It may even seem tempting for parents to delay the introduction of solid foods until a baby has a full set of teeth and enough motor control to feed himself, but in fact the addition of solids foods at six months (as a supplement to ongoing breastfeeding) is a necessary step toward healthy growth and development.[3] After six months of age, exclusive breastfeeding falls short of a few key nutrients necessary to support a child's continued growth.[4] For this reason, pediatric health agencies in most countries around the world recommend introducing solid foods between 4 and 6 months of age while continuing to supplement the child's diet with breast milk for the first year of life, or longer if desired.[5,6]

With all of the uncertainty new parents feel about when, what, how, and how much to feed their babies, it helps to remember that human infants come into this world hardwired to grow into solid-food eaters. Throughout history, parents all over the world had little choice but to feed their babies with appropriately

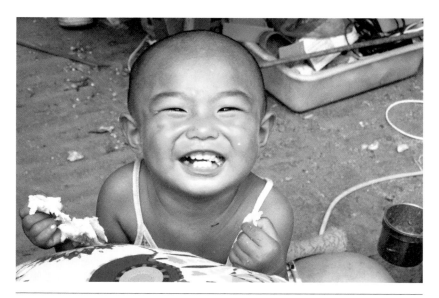

Figure 3.1   Throughout history, children have been fed modified versions of the same foods eaten by their parents.

modified versions of the *very same foods* the parents were eating. In this way, local eating cultures and cuisines were passed from generation to generation.

Since the mid-1900s when parents began to rely more on infant formula in many parts of the world, we simultaneously became more reliant on the baby food industry, in general, to dictate the best first foods for our offspring. The widespread availability and successful marketing of commercial baby foods have made early feeding more convenient for busy parents. However, there is a potential downside to this convenience. Firstly, relying on refined, commercial baby foods can effectively set an early precedent for "The Kids' Menu." Children who become accustomed to a narrow range of flavors in early childhood may struggle to accept new or unfamiliar foods later in childhood. Studies exploring the factors that affect a child's acceptance of vegetables, for example, suggest that early, repeated exposure to such foods is important.[7,8] Parental modeling of a healthful, varied diet also appears to be key. For the most part, the flavors children are exposed to early in life set the foundation for flavor preferences later on. The second drawback of relying on commercially prepared baby food is that our global shift toward convenience foods has left many parents feeling insecure about one of our most instinctive human skills: the ability to prepare and provide food for our own offspring.

CASE STUDY 3.1

Aisha is a 28-year-old mother of a healthy, happy, five-month-old boy named Neal. As she nears the end of her maternity leave from the university where she works full-time as a senior administrative assistant, Aisha is feeling ready to go back to work. The university has a lovely daycare facility where she can leave her son while she is at work and she plans to begin transitioning him to solid foods, so that she can leave both pumped breast milk and solid foods for the daycare teachers to feed Neal during the day. (The office building where she works also has a special room for lactating mothers to use, so Aisha can pump milk as needed and store it in the refrigerator for later.)

On the morning that she decides to start feeding Neal solid foods, she finds herself at the supermarket, staring at a wall full of boxes of infant cereal and little glass jars, containing an enormous variety of different packaged infant foods. Each colorful little jar and box has a happy, healthy baby pictured somewhere on the front. For years, Aisha has walked by this shelf, subconsciously internalizing the images of those happy babies and the colorful vegetables inside the jars, so she doesn't think twice about where to get her baby's first solid meal. She decides to start Neal on white rice cereal, then sweet potatoes. At first, Neal spits out the unfamiliar food and struggles to coordinate his tongue so that the mashed food actually gets to the back of his throat where he can swallow it. But after a week, he's getting better at it and more of the solid food is ending up in his stomach, instead of on his highchair table—or the kitchen floor.

A few weeks later, Aisha is preparing a special sweet potato dish that her husband remembers eating as a child when his family celebrated Rosh Hashanah. She wonders whether it would be okay to let Neal try some of this. But is it safe?

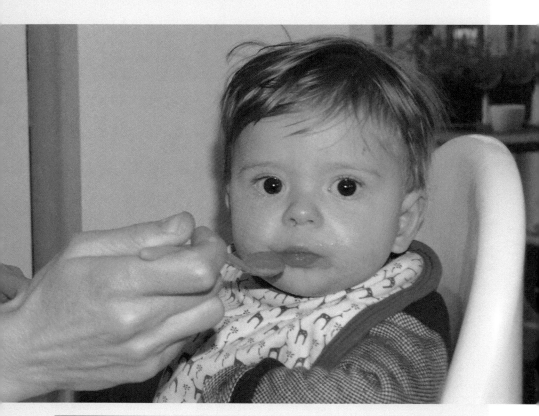

Figure 3.2 First foods provide an opportunity to begin passing on family traditions.

Are babies allowed to have real sweet potatoes? What about the olive oil she added …? Is that safe for babies? Aisha calls her mother to ask if she knows the answer to these questions and her mother laughs, "My dear, you grew up in a time and place where there were no baby food jars. You ate what we ate—with a little less spice. We blended cooked vegetables that had been sautéed in olive oil with onions and garlic … . When you were a year old, we were already adding a little bit of chili to your foods, so you would get used to the flavors we enjoyed eating. To this day, I think one of the reasons you enjoy the tastes of so many different cuisines is that we exposed you to many different flavors when you were young."

Aisha hangs up the phone and puts a tablespoon of the sweet potato mash into a small bowl. She mashes it a bit more and adds some breast milk until the consistency looks like it will be manageable for Neal. At first taste, he looks at her questioningly and immediately spits out the new flavor. After a small pause, she sees him licking his lips to get the flavor back for a second taste. She offers him another spoon, smaller this time, and he seems to keep the food in his mouth for a moment before swallowing it. By the fourth spoonful, Neal is opening his mouth like a baby bird for the next bite. The next day, Neal's father is delighted to learn that his son shares his love of his family's own version of *tzimmes*.

Aisha decides to make a larger batch of this homemade baby food and she freezes it in a covered ice cube tray, so that she can quickly reheat it as needed on the days she doesn't have time to cook fresh baby food. She starts doing this with a variety of vegetables as she's preparing them for the adults to eat and soon, she has an impressive repertoire of "Neal meals" that are convenient and less expensive than the baby food jars she was buying at the store. Neal is now six years old—a happy first-grader, who's also an adventurous eater. His mother's sweet potato mash will always be one of his favorites!

ARE YOU READY FOR THIS?

How does a parent know when her baby is developmentally ready to begin eating solid foods? In addition to showing interest in foods, babies who are getting ready to eat solids will also begin to demonstrate some new skills. Somewhere between 5 and 8 months, a baby learns to sit up, at first with some help, and eventually independently. By this age, they've also begun to master the art of head control. (Remember that a baby's head is relatively heavy for them in the early months, when compared with the weight of their bodies.) Mastering head control means that the baby can turn toward food and eventually open and guide their mouths toward spoons in the vicinity. While newborns will reflexively spit substances out by pushing forward with their tongues, most 6- to 8-month-olds will have the coordination to draw food into their mouths, first by using their lips to scrape food off the spoon and secondly by moving soft solids to the back of the tongue where it can be mashed further and eventually swallowed. You've probably never given any real thought to the complexity of the coordination involved in the chewing and swallowing of food. After all, we do it every day without even thinking about it. But babies who are getting ready to begin eating solid foods are also getting ready to learn a brand new set of motor patterns and skills. It can be an exciting (and messy) time for everyone involved. If parents keep in mind just how challenging it is for their little one to learn this new skills set, they'll be less likely to get frustrated and lose their sense of humor—an essential ingredient for a good solid meal!

WHAT ARE THE BEST FIRST FOODS?

Once a child has reached an appropriate age and begins to show signs of developmental readiness for solid feeding, the first question that usually arises is, What foods should we start with? What foods are safe and nutritious for a first-time eater? Refined white rice cereal is still recommended by many pediatricians in developed countries because it is free of the common food allergens, usually fortified with iron, and thought to be easy to digest. However, the refined nature of white rice cereal means that it is also quickly converted into simple sugars by the body. These sugars enter the bloodstream quickly, leading to spikes of glucose and insulin in the blood that may not be healthy for babies in the long term. For this reason, some pediatricians feel that refined white rice cereal is a suboptimal choice for baby's first meal and suggest starting with pureed vegetables instead. The fiber in vegetables, especially unrefined or homemade baby purees, slows the entry of glucose into the blood, lowering the glycemic index of the food, which stabilizes blood sugar levels and delays the return of hunger. In general, babies can safely eat most fruits and vegetables, perhaps starting with milder flavors like baked sweet potatoes, avocados, peas, and bananas, and gradually adding variety as each new food is successfully introduced and tolerated.

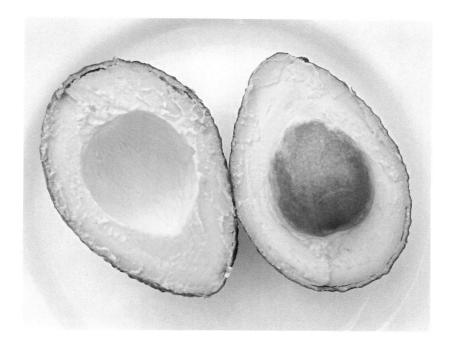

Figure 3.3   Mashed or pureed avocado, baked sweet potatoes, peas and bananas are some examples of good first foods.

In selecting foods for their baby, the guiding principle for parents should be to build up to a diet that includes a *variety* of foods.[9] Variety maximizes the breadth of nutrients provided by the solid portion of a baby's diet. It may be best to feed each vegetable separately to an emerging eater, rather than offering vegetable purees that incorporate a blend of different vegetables into a single serving. There are two reasons for this: Firstly, as babies begin learning to identify the taste, smell, color, and flavor of each new food, it can be confusing when they are presented with multi-vegetable blends, at least in the early weeks of solid feeding. Secondly, it's easier to identify the cause of any potential food intolerance when new foods are presented separately. In general, a good diet for a healthy baby encompasses a variety of wholesome vegetables, fruits, and whole grains in addition to sufficient iron-containing foods.

First Tastes Around the World

There is no hard science that explicitly states which first foods are best and, in fact, the enormous variation in first foods routinely fed to babies around the world indicates that babies can thrive on a wide range of first foods. Often, these foods reflect the eating traditions of each specific country as well as taking the form of a ritual or blessing. In Japan, the tradition of Okuizome (first meal) takes place somewhere between 100 and 120 days after birth. This first meal contains a variety of foods including sticky rice, fish, octopus, and pickled vegetables, and symbolizes the abundance that Japanese parents wish their children to enjoy throughout their lives. In Kenya, sweet potatoes are commonly given as a first food. Rich in fiber, vitamin A, and other important nutrients, this is a sensible choice for promoting the good health of babies in the region. Jamaican babies are treated to first foods consisting of locally grown tropical fruits, like papaya,

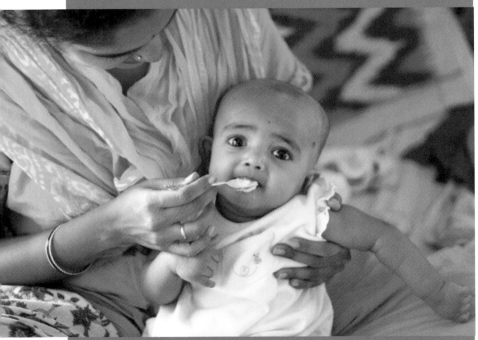

Figure 3.4   Annaprasana is the Hindu ritual first meal, during which babies are fed rice porridge that has been blessed by older family members.

banana, and mango, while their counterparts in China are introduced to rice dishes mixed with small amounts of fish, carrots, seaweed, and eggs. Vietnamese babies are fed a traditional soup, flavored with fish sauce and shrimp, for their first meal, while Swedish parents mix up *välling*, a wheat-based porridge made with powdered milk and palm oil. The French approach feeding (throughout childhood) as part of a child's formal education, carefully exposing children to a wide variety of healthful foods in order to cultivate a refined palate. French babies are routinely fed things like leek soup, creamed spinach, and pureed cauliflower for their first culinary adventures.

What do all of these first foods have in common? They reflect the rich cultural heritage and, to some extent, the values of any given society. For example, many American parents value the convenience of ready-made baby foods over the importance of educating the palate that French parents might see as a priority. These cultural differences subtly shape our children's preferences and, with them, our children's health. However, the eating culture of any given family can trump that of the society in which they live, especially when it comes to decisions about infant feeding. While children are young, parents have a tremendous window of opportunity to expose their offspring to a variety of healthful food choices, thereby programming their palates to prefer foods that are good for them. Parents around the world should be encouraged to choose first foods that reflect their unique values and their family's heritage—while simultaneously supporting the long-term health and wellbeing of the next generation.

IMPORTANT NUTRIENTS FOR GROWING BODIES

First foods are sometimes called complementary foods because they're intended to complement breast milk in a baby's diet. Iron reserves begin to deplete around six months of age, so complementary foods that provide a good source of iron are excellent choices. Spinach, green peas, apricots, and prunes are all examples of iron-containing complementary foods. Well-cooked and pureed legumes like chick peas, white beans, kidney beans, black beans, or lentils are also good sources of iron and can be incorporated into a healthy baby's diet. In general, the iron found in meats is more easily absorbed by the body, so small amounts of sustainably raised meats, chicken, and fish can also be cooked and pureed for babies, usually from about eight or nine months of age onward. For parents who choose to introduce animal-based proteins like meats, the recommended age for introducing these foods varies from country to country, so this is another instance where parents should use their best judgment and carefully observe their own child to assess her readiness. Despite being somewhat less efficiently absorbed, plant sources of iron may have other health benefits and several studies have shown that pairing a good source of vitamin C with meals containing either plant or meat sources of iron can help to increase the amount of iron that is absorbed. Adding a source of vitamin C, like a side of pureed orange, kiwi, or melon, may help to facilitate iron absorption.

Calcium is another important nutrient for growth in babies and young children. This mineral supports growth, maintenance, and repair of bones and teeth, among other important functions. Luckily, both breast milk and infant formula provide plenty of calcium for a healthy, growing child. (See the note in Chapter 2 for more information on vitamin D supplementation during exclusive breastfeeding in certain parts of the world.)

In developing counties, a third nutrient is very important for maintaining the health of babies and older children. This nutrient is vitamin A, which is important for protecting eyesight and preventing night blindness, but it's also life-saving in parts of the world where children are particularly vulnerable to infections—especially when those children also more likely to be undernourished. In under-resourced parts of the world, a small dose of vitamin A, given by mouth every six months at a local health clinic, can save a child's life. Vitamin A is found in a variety of orange fruits and vegetables (sweet potato, carrots, butternut squash, and apricots) as well as dark green vegetables (spinach, kale, broccoli, collards).

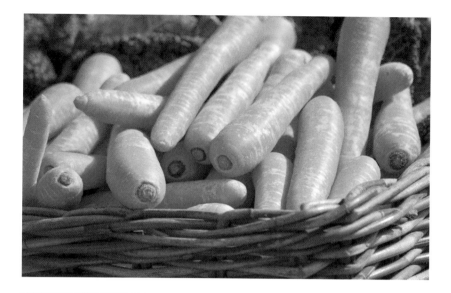

Figure 3.5 Orange vegetables are an excellent source of vitamin A.

Eat the Rainbow

When we choose vegetables and fruits of many different colors, we are automatically maximizing the nutrient diversity of our meals. Different colors of fresh produce are associated with different nutrient profiles, so instead of trying to memorize which vegetable contains which vitamins, the simple principle of eating the rainbow will help keep the nutrient needs of the entire family covered. Every day, children and adults should try to enjoy at least five servings of fruits or vegetables—ideally including a variety of colors! Not only will this maximize the spectrum of nutrients a child receives, but it will also minimize her exposure to any potential toxins or other harmful substances (like pesticide residues) that may be present in trace amounts in food. Eating a varied diet is also more likely to satisfy hunger as well as food cravings that could be brought on by nutrient deficiencies.

FOODS TO AVOID DURING THE FIRST YEAR

There are certain foods that are best avoided during a child's first year of life. Feeding these foods to a baby can increase the risk of foodborne illnesses or cause digestive difficulties. These foods include:

1. **Honey.** Honey can contain botulism spores, which if ingested by an adult or older child would almost certainly not cause disease. However, botulism spores can germinate in the immature intestines of a baby and cause serious illness. Corn syrup poses a similar risk and should also be avoided in children under one year of age.
2. **Home-canned foods.** Low-acid, home-canned foods (such as meat, poultry, fish, green beans, carrots, and asparagus) can also carry botulism. If a family eats these foods, it may be wise to avoid serving them to babies. If home-canned foods are a staple of the family diet, parents should be encouraged to discuss this with a pediatrician and consult with a reputable home-canning agency.
3. **Milk.** Milk, other than breast milk or infant formula, including cow's, goat's, soy, rice, and almond milks, can be difficult for babies to digest in their first year of life. They're also nutritionally inadequate for infants, who still depend on the wide variety of nutrients present in breast or formula milk. Milk products other than breast milk and infant formula can be introduced gradually after a year of age.
4. **What about common food allergens?** Historically, research suggested that delaying or entirely avoiding certain highly allergenic foods (e.g., peanuts, milk, egg whites, wheat, and shellfish), especially for babies with a family history of allergies, was a recommended approach to preventing the later development of food allergies in children. However, more recent research suggests that avoiding early exposure to common food allergens may not significantly reduce a child's risk of developing food allergies.[10,11] Parents who are concerned about exposing their child to potential food allergens should consult a pediatrician for an individualized assessment of the relative risks and benefits of avoiding these foods.
5. **Fish contaminated with mercury.** Over the last decade, regulatory groups including the FDA and the EPA have warned that it may be wise to limit a young child's intake of fish that could potentially contain elevated levels of mercury. Some of the fish that should be avoided or

limited in a baby's diet are shark, swordfish, king mackerel, tilefish, and white albacore tuna (different from canned, light tuna).[12] See Chapter 10 on environmental sustainability and health for more details.

6. **High-sugar and/or high-salt foods.** It may seem intuitive to most parents that babies and children should not be fed foods that are high in salt or added sugar. However, excessive amounts of salt and sugar are commonly added to many foods that are marketed to children. (See Chapter 7 on food marketing.) So, it's worth reminding parents about the value of exposing young children to the natural flavors of real foods instead of the highly processed versions of those foods. For example, homemade baked or steamed potatoes, perhaps mashed with a bit of real butter, are likely to be much lower in salt and unhealthy fats than are french fries from a fast food restaurant. Homemade oatmeal, even with a bit of maple syrup, is likely far lower in sugar than processed, sweetened cereals that are marketed to children all over the world. Again, a recurring theme emerges: when foods are prepared for a child by someone who has a vested interest in the long-term health of that child, the foods will more likely be healthful and contain only reasonable amounts of fat, sugar, and salt. When parents and loving caregivers take the job of feeding children into their own hands, they are more likely to set their children up for a lifetime of healthful eating.

Parent Forum

The Power of Moderation

As the US holiday season approaches, my excitement about the upcoming festivities is sometimes mixed with a little uncertainty. Halloween, Diwali, Thanksgiving, Hanukkah, Christmas: whatever you celebrate, you probably know that this time of year usually involves a whole lot of eating—and a seemingly endless stream of treats. If you happen to live in the US, those treats are likely to be super-sized, adding another layer of complexity to the challenge of eating sensibly. For our family, with its unusual set of Indian, German, and Jewish South African roots, the holiday season seems particularly out of control because we celebrate all of the above holidays, one after another.

At this time of year, I'm reminded of how important it is to teach our children the art of moderation. My message to them is simple: bigger is not always better. We can enjoy absolutely any food, as long as it's consumed in moderation. A small piece of chocolate eaten after a nutritious meal and before a good tooth brushing? Okay. A king-size KitKat, scarfed down in front of the TV with a Coke and a packet of Doritos? Houston, we have a problem. We live in a country of seemingly limitless opportunity. From a young age, we learn that if we can dream it, we can build it! If it already exists, we can make it bigger—and add cheese. Don't get me wrong: I love the spirit of thinking big here in the US, but one thing we haven't yet learned is that, when it comes to our food, less really would be more for most people. When we eat smaller amounts of higher quality food, we maximize our enjoyment of one of life's great pleasures: eating! Michael Pollan advises us to "spend more, eat less" so we don't end up breaking the bank on more-expensive, higher-quality food. The truth is that when we eat real, fresh food in modest amounts (even if it's cooked with a pat of butter and a sprinkle of salt), it doesn't take much to leave us feeling completely satisfied. In contrast, when we overindulge on poor-quality, low-nutrient foods, our bodies are left feeling cheated—and worse yet, guilty for overindulging!

If our children grow up understanding that no food is forbidden, as long as the *amount* they eat is reasonable, we set them free to really enjoy their food—holiday treats and all!

Here are some small changes that can help turn every meal feel into a guilt-free indulgence.

1. **The half trick.** The next time you or your children see something in a bakery window that looks irresistible, go ahead. Buy that chocolate croissant, cut it in half before you sit down, and pack the other half in a paper bag for tomorrow. Tuck it away, where it won't be seen. Then enjoy your perfectly reasonable treat. The half trick is great for eating at restaurants, too! Consider ordering a to-go container to arrive with your meal, and box up half of everything before you start eating.

2. **Sit down.** When you're eating, sit at a table and make sure there are NO screens to distract you. Then, focus on the taste of your food by eating a little bit more slowly and perhaps pausing between each bite. You'll actually feel like you've eaten more than you have!

3. **Buy smaller plates and glasses.** A small plate makes the food on it look more plentiful and your stomach is more likely to tell you you've

had enough after the first serving. Researchers have actually proven that we eat more when we use bigger plates. The same rule applies to glasses! (Many hardware stores carry very affordable, sturdy dishes that are smaller than fancy ones at designer stores.)

4. **The power of the healthy alternative.** Having delicious (healthier) alternatives on hand — like crunchy vegetables with homemade dips or dressings, fresh or dried fruits, and nuts — makes it easier to make better choices most of the time.

5. **Actions speak louder than words.** When kids see that their parents are able to enjoy a small treat on occasion—and then stop—they learn a great lesson: Less is more. A small treat, enjoyed guilt-free because the amount is right, is a true luxury. After all, that's how treats were meant to be eaten.

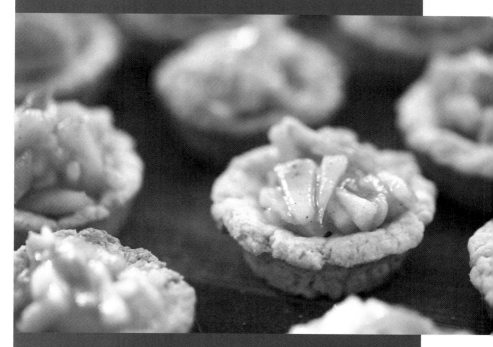

Figure 3.6   Homemade treats are almost always more nutritious than packaged alternatives—and we have more control over their size!

6. **Go for homemade.** Homemade treats are the best kind, by far. When we bake our own cakes, cookies, and other goodies, the moderation is built right in. First, the ingredients we use will almost certainly be more nutritious (and fresher) than any packaged items. And unlike the makers of packaged foods, we care about the health of the people who are going to be eating those foods, so we'll automatically go easy on the fat, sugar, and salt. Finally, baking treats from scratch takes time and effort. This fact has a rate-limiting effect that naturally regulates the frequency of our indulgences.

Food should be enjoyed every day—and at every meal. By giving our children the gift of moderation, they'll always remember that good things really do come in smaller packages.

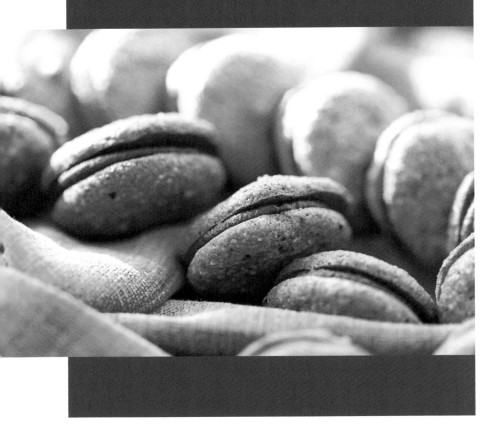

CHAPTER 4

HOW FOOD HELPS CHILDREN GROW: TEACHING KIDS TO LOVE THE FOODS THAT LOVE THEM BACK

From birth until the teenage years, our children are involved in two high-intensity, interrelated activities called growth and development. In less than two decades, a tiny, helpless newborn will be transformed into an almost fully grown adult. Like most diseases, malnutrition (either under- or over-nutrition) will interfere with the normal processes involved in healthy growth and development. On the other hand, balanced nutrition throughout childhood and adolescence can set a child up for lifelong good health and a preference for health-promoting foods.

How do we measure growth and development? The term *growth* usually refers to increases in three categories: weight, height (or length in babies), and head circumference. These three parameters are the ones pediatricians use to assess growth through the practice of growth monitoring. Measured values for height, weight, and head circumference are recorded and plotted on a growth chart at regular time intervals and the trends that emerge are then examined for consistency and compared with a range of normal values, averaged from many healthy babies over their growth periods. Evaluating and tracking a child's growth over time in this way can provide important information about the child's wellbeing. For example, a sudden drop-off in weight may indicate an acute illness, while failure to grow in height may be a sign of chronic disease,

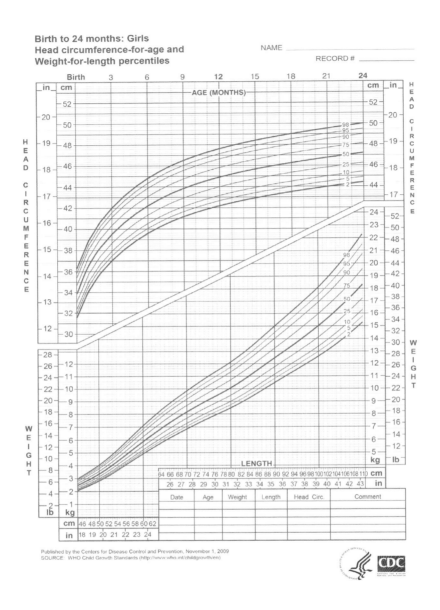

Figure 4.1   Example of a growth chart for girls 0-24 months of age.

including long-standing malnutrition. In parts of the world where obesity and overweight are more prevalent in children, growth monitoring can help physicians assess and track a child's weight and make recommendations for changes in eating behavior and physical activity.

Closely related to growth, a child's development can also be impacted by the quality of her diet. Development refers to the progressive acquisition of age-appropriate skills or characteristics and it can occur with or without changes in size. For example, walking and talking are developmental milestones that occur during the first and second years of life, which are also periods of rapid physical growth. Pubertal development occurs later, during adolescence, and may occur independently of changes in height or weight.

Both growth and development are processes that are highly dependent on adequate nutrition. Yet, there are a host of environmental factors that can undermine the quality of a child's diet from birth through adolescence. These factors range from socioeconomic considerations that can limit access to healthful foods to educational factors, including the parents' level of understanding about what makes up a balanced meal. Even cultural factors can influence the

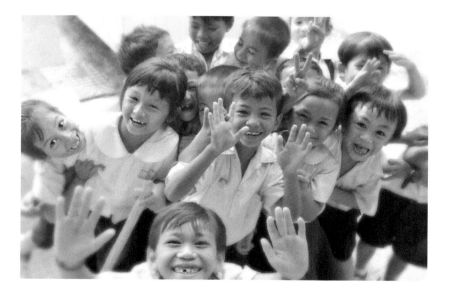

Figure 4.2   Growth and Development are interrelated processes that are highly dependent on adequate nutrition.

quality of nutrition a child receives. In many parts of the world, cultural beliefs about the relative value of male versus female children have historically led to epidemics of under-nutrition (and even infanticide) among girls.

Reshaping misguided cultural beliefs and eradicating widespread resource shortages are complicated tasks, and not ones that can be adequately addressed in a child nutrition guide, but we can try to improve the level of understanding among parents and caregivers about what makes up a balanced meal. Even in profoundly under-resourced areas, most parents will subtly reallocate resources to support the health of their children, if they're given the right information to guide those health-promoting shifts. So, let's start by discussing what we know about the components of food and how our children's bodies use these parts to protect their health and promote their successful growth and development.

MEET THE NUTRIENTS

Before we launch into a discussion about carbohydrates, proteins, fats, vitamins, and minerals (and how much of each of these our children need to grow), let's go back to basics and talk briefly about three of the most critical components of a healthy child's diet. In order to grow, thrive, and maintain a healthy weight, our children need to consume an adequate amount of fresh vegetables, fresh fruits, and water. The reason for giving these foods special emphasis has to do with the widespread shifts in eating that have happened in recent decades. The increasing availability of highly processed foods, including sweetened drinks, has put immense pressure on our children's health. Making space in our children's meals for these critical components—water and plants—may well be the most important thing we can do for their health in the twenty-first century and beyond. Research has repeatedly underscored the importance of adequate fruit and vegetable consumption in protecting our health and the health of our children.[1-3] In the US, on average, a child eats too few fruits and vegetables and drinks too many sweetened beverages.[4-6] Michael Pollan, a highly respected journalist and professor of nutrition science at the University of California at Berkeley, simplified this advice in his seven-word description of what we should be eating to optimize our health:

Eat food. Not too much. Mostly plants.

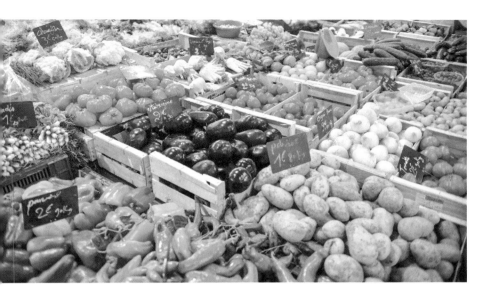

Figure 4.3 Consuming adequate amounts of vegetables, fresh fruits and water may be the most important objective of a healthy diet for children growing up in the 21st century.

If we can keep Pollan's sensible advice in mind as we define our goals for feeding our children, we can teach them to love the foods that will "love them back" by helping to protect their health for a lifetime.

This advice is certainly not meant to suggest that a child should live on fruits, vegetables, and water alone. In order to have the energy to fuel growth, repair tissues, power physical activities, and support neurological development, a child also needs a variety of other foods, including those that provide adequate amounts of three macronutrients: carbohydrates, proteins, and fats.

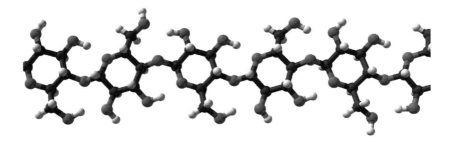

Figure 4.4   Polysaccharides are made up of single sugar units, linked together by chemical bonds.

CARBOHYDRATES

Dietary carbohydrates include foods that are rich in starch or sugar. The chemical name for starch is polysaccharide ("poly" meaning *many* and "saccharide" meaning *sugars*). The many sugars that make up a complex carbohydrate are linked by chemical bonds that must be broken down by the body during the process of digestion. The other major sub-category of carbohydrates (the kind we often tend to over-consume) is the simple carbohydrates, otherwise known as simple sugars. Simple sugars are one- or two-unit sugars (mono- or disaccharides) that are more quickly and easily digested and absorbed by the body. While this may sound like a good thing at first, the overconsumption of simple sugars can have serious negative consequences for our health and the health of our children.

Sugar: Too Much of a Good Thing

The overconsumption of sugar has become a major health problem for children and adults in many parts of the world. Because of this, sugar has sometimes been referred to as a toxin, especially in the US, where consumption rates are highest. While our bodies need a small amount of sugar to fuel the brain, the excessive consumption of sugar can certainly have a toxic effect on our bodies. In many parts of the world, changes in the culture of eating have made it increasingly difficult to avoid over-consuming sugar. Excess sugar is converted to fat, causing overweight and obesity.[7] Eating too much sugar is also associated with a higher risk of developing insulin resistance and type 2 diabetes.[7,8] In the developing world, where dental caries (cavities) are a major problem for many children, this public health concern is severely aggravated by increasing rates of sugar consumption.[9,10]

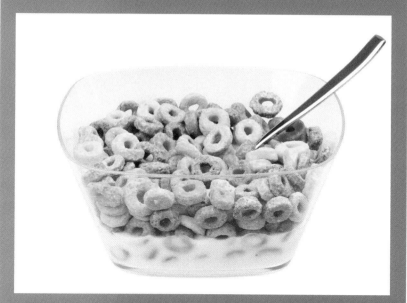

Figure 4.5 Most of the excess sugar in our children's diets comes from processed foods, like sweetened breakfast cereals.

Surprisingly, that major source of simple sugar in our children's diets isn't usually the sugar bowl on the table. Most of the excess sugar in the contemporary child's diet comes from processed foods, including breakfast cereals, and sodas and other sweetened beverages. Packaged foods often have large amounts of sugar added to increase their palatability (making us want them more) and to increase their shelf life because additives like corn syrup act as a preservative. For these reasons, even items like packaged bread and bottled salad dressings will often have some form of simple sugar added to them. This is especially true in the US where corn subsidies have made corn syrup extremely inexpensive for processed food manufacturers.

This trend has made the moderate consumption of sugar a difficult task to accomplish. One way to try to achieve this lofty goal—the moderate consumption of sugar—is to cook at home using mostly fresh, whole ingredients. When a parent or loving caregiver bakes a cake for a child's birthday celebration, the baker has control over how much sugar goes into the final product. By making homemade treats, which are served to children occasionally (not daily), parents can protect their children's health and teach them the art of moderation.

The simplest and most ubiquitous of the simple sugars is glucose, a single-unit sugar that our bodies can break down to make energy or convert into body energy stores, including fat. A close relative of this sugar is fructose, the kind of sugar found in fruits, as well as many other foods. When glucose and fructose are linked together, they form another kind of simple carbohydrate, the disaccharide called sucrose, which is also known as table sugar. Another well-known disaccharide is the two-unit sugar called lactose. Lactose is the disaccharide found in milk and dairy products. Around the world, there are individuals and entire communities who cannot easily digest lactose—a condition known as lactose intolerance. When lactose-intolerant individuals ingest dairy products, the undigested lactose molecules pass through the gut, where they are consumed by gas-producing bacteria. This commonly leads to symptoms like abdominal bloating, distention, and severe discomfort.

Side note: Historically, many cultures have seen cow's milk as an invaluable source of calcium for growing children. While cow's milk is an excellent source of this important nutrient, there are many other good sources of dietary calcium, including dark green leafy vegetables, canned fish with bones, yogurt, cheese, and fortified nut milks.

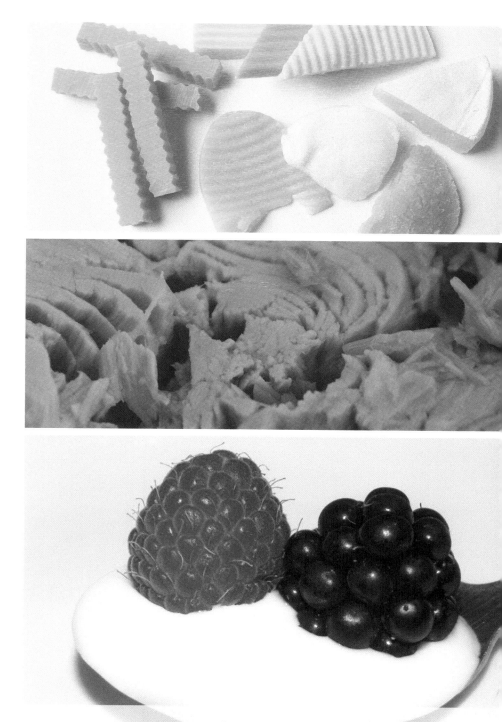

Figure 4.6 Cheese, canned fish with bones, and yoghurt are calcium-rich foods.

Unlike the one- or two-unit sugars associated with the family of simple carbohydrates, complex carbohydrates are made up of many glucose molecules linked together by chemical bonds. Starchy foods, like potatoes, bread, pasta, and rice are high in complex carbohydrates. Dietary fiber is also a form of complex carbohydrate. The major difference is that dietary fiber provides little or no energy (calories) because our bodies cannot break down the bonds between the single sugar units in this kind of complex carbohydrate. Additionally, there are two subtypes of dietary fiber. Soluble fiber dissolves in water and supports the health of the intestinal walls. Insoluble fiber absorbs water (like a sponge) and acts as a stool softener, speeding up the passage of food through the intestinal tract. This prevents constipation, a common problem in children who eat a diet that is high in refined (low-fiber) carbohydrates. Both types of fiber are found in fruits and vegetables. The carbohydrates in a child's diet should ideally be unrefined, to support intestinal health and maximize nutrient density. This means choosing whole-grain breads over white breads and brown rice over white rice whenever possible. Unrefined carbohydrates take longer to digest so they also sustain a child's satiety, delaying the return of hunger and helping to stabilize blood sugar levels.

The Glycemic Index

The glycemic index of a food is the measure of the speed at which glucose enters the bloodstream after eating it. Sodas and candy, for example, are high in simple sugars like sucrose and glucose. After eating these, the body is able to quickly digest and absorb the glucose in these foods, leading to a sizable spike in blood sugar levels. The body responds by releasing large amounts of insulin, the hormone responsible for lowering blood sugar levels. Because the vigorous insulin response to the spike in blood glucose is reactive, the response results in a period of time when blood sugar levels may actually fall into the lower range of normal.[11] This dip in blood sugar leads to the sensation of hunger and explains why a child can feel hungry soon after eating a snack that's high in simple sugars. This physiological phenomenon can even occur in babies who are fed highly processed baby foods, like refined baby cereals, because refined cereals have a relatively high glycemic index.

In general, meals and snacks that contain fiber, protein, and/or healthy fats are far better choices for sustaining satiety or delaying the return of hunger. Brown rice and whole-wheat bread, for example, have lower

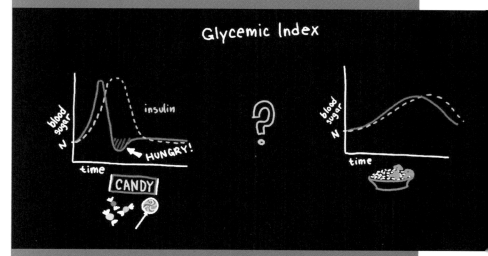

Figure 4.7 When glucose enters the blood quickly, the vigorous insulin response can cause fluctuations in blood sugar that lead to the early return of hunger.

glycemic indexes than white rice and white bread have. Sensible, low-glycemic snacks, like a slice of cheese with a whole-grain cracker, an avocado and tomato sandwich on whole-grain bread, or a handful of raw and unsalted almonds will stabilize blood sugar levels much more effectively than snacks like potato chips and sweetened drinks. Because of the associated fiber, whole fruits are sensible treats with a lower glycemic index than are candy bars or processed, sugary desserts.

PROTEIN

Proteins are another important part of a healthy child's diet. These foods help to support the growth and repair of all body tissues as well as performing a variety of important regulatory roles. Proteins are critical to supporting the functioning of the immune system, transporting oxygen, as well as maintaining fluid balance in the body. In a growing child's body, proteins can be thought of as the building blocks and they are made up of subunits called amino acids. There are twenty different kinds of amino acids and the human body can synthesize them to some extent. However, nine of those twenty are called "essential amino acids" because our bodies cannot make enough of them to support optimal health. For this reason, we rely on food to provide us with these essential nutrients. Protein-rich foods can come from animal sources, including eggs, fish, chicken, and red meat. Dairy products like yogurt and cheese are also good sources of protein. But they can also be found in plant-based foods, like tofu, nuts, beans, and lentils. An important distinction between these different sources of protein is that animal sources of protein tend to be complete, meaning that they contain all of the essential nutrients in adequate amounts to support growth, maintenance, and repair of body tissues. Plant-based proteins tend to be incomplete, meaning that they must be combined with other foods in order to support optimal health. Luckily, many traditional food combinations were designed to pair complementary sources of amino acids. In Mexico, for example, beans and rice are a staple combination, delivering a complete set of amino acids. In India, lentils and rice are another example of a food pairing that serves as a complete protein source for growing children. It's important to note that plant-based sources of protein may have other important benefits for our children's health (and our own). Plant-based proteins tend to be higher in fiber and lower in cholesterol and saturated fat than animal products. They are also usually more economical and can help families stay healthy when the food budget is tight. As with all diets, increasing the variety of plant-based protein sources in a vegetarian diet will almost certainly support the nutrient needs of a growing vegetarian child.

The Downside of the Single-nutrient Solution

In many parts of the developed world, people consume much more animal-based protein than they need—sometimes to the point where it's detrimental to their health. In cultures where excess nutrition and obesity are more common problems than food shortage is, we tend to see a pendulum effect when it comes to our diets. For example, in the 80s and early 90s, avoiding fat consumption became a central dietary goal, influencing many of our dietary recommendations. As the fat was taken out of many foods, like yogurts and breakfast cereals, more sugar was added to increase the palatability of the fat-free foods so that they would continue to sell. At the same time, the widespread availability of cheap corn syrups in the US meant that the consumption of simple carbohydrates skyrocketed as the general public tried to reduce their intake of fats. Paradoxically, obesity rates in the US increased during this same time period, so researchers began to focus on sugar as a potential culprit. There is no doubt that the enormous amount of sugar in the Western diet has contributed to the obesity epidemic. However, we must be careful not to repeat the mistakes of the past. Some food writers and nutritionists are now suggesting that we should severely decrease our intake of all carbohydrates, including unrefined, complex carbohydrates (the "good carbs"). Instead, the proponents of the extremely low-carb diet seem to suggest that diets high in animal protein could be the solution to our modern epidemics of obesity and diabetes. The danger, of course, is that the pendulum swings to the extreme and that there are unforeseen health consequences that could once again negatively affect the health of entire populations.

Throughout history, the diets that have best supported human health and longevity have been balanced, moderate diets that included a variety of real, minimally processed foods, prepared in diverse and interesting ways to maximize flavor. These are also the diets that have withstood the test of time because they've sufficiently varied to sustain our enjoyment of food. We are hardwired to enjoy our food, so restrictive diets that focus on eliminating a single macronutrient in favor of another are destined to fail. When it comes to our children's food, one of our greatest responsibilities is to leave the next generation with a love of the foods that will simultaneously support their health and their enjoyment of food.

FATS

Dietary fats have been a major topic of discussion (and confusion) in recent decades. Fats perform several important functions that are critical for the healthy growth and development of a child. They support brain development and the functioning of the nervous system, they protect and cushion vital internal organs, they form an important energy storage reservoir, and they help maintain correct body temperature by insulating us. In addition, when children consume a meal that contains an appropriate amount of fat, they're less likely to feel hungry soon afterwards because fat actually lowers the glycemic index of the food.[11]

WHAT IS "HEALTHY FAT"?

Dietary fats can be divided into two main categories: saturated and unsaturated fats. Saturated fats get their name from the fact that their fatty acids are relatively straight and flat so they can pack together densely. Because of this, saturated fats are usually solids at room temperature. Examples of saturated fats are butter and the solid, white fat found in meats.

Unsaturated fats can be divided into two types. Naturally occurring unsaturated fats are usually liquids at room temperature (like olive oil) because their fatty acids are kinked in ways that make it difficult for them to stack together into a solid structure. However, these fatty acids can be chemically altered so that they will stay solid at room temperature. The synthetic unsaturated fats used to make most margarines have been altered in this way. Chemically altered unsaturated fats are also used to make oils that can be reheated and used for commercial deep frying—like the oils used in french fry machines. Synthetic, or chemically altered, unsaturated fats are inherently unstable, so temperature changes, like those that occur when they are repeatedly reheated, generate a new kind of fat called trans fat.

In recent decades, dietary fats (especially saturated fats and trans fats) have been implicated in the development of heart disease, specifically because of their role in forming plaques in the arteries.[12-14] More recently, researchers have suggested that in trying to prevent heart disease, the types of fat consumed may be more important than the total amount of fat consumed. Replacing saturated fats with naturally occurring unsaturated ones may be better for our health than simply reducing total fat consumption.[15] Once again, the moderate consumption of a variety of healthful foods appears to be the best way to support our health and the health of our children.

WATER

We often forget to talk about water when we're discussing the components of a healthy diet or a healthy meal. One possible reason for this glaring omission is the simple fact that, in many parts of the world, including the US, water is free so we don't (yet) have a powerful commercial water industry, poised to ensure its consumption. Indeed, some people would argue that America's cultural focus on the importance of drinking milk is, to some extent, the result of a thriving dairy industry. If adequate amounts of calcium-containing foods are consumed throughout the day, a child usually does not need to drink milk with every meal. Regular hydration with water, however, is critically important. Our bodies are made up of approximately 50% water and, without it, we would die more quickly than we would if we were to be starved of food. Maintaining homeostasis—the state of physiological equilibrium that the body strives for—is highly dependent on the availability of water. Clean, safe water is the ideal drink for a healthy child—both as a thirst quencher and to accompany any meal. While the absolute amount of water that a child needs each day depends on several factors (including climate, activity level, and body size), endorsing water as the default drink for healthy children is almost always a good idea.

SALT

Like sugar, the salt content of our diets has increased dramatically in recent years, especially in parts of the world where we've begun to rely heavily on processed food. There is no question that on average in the US, a child today consumes too much salt (or dietary sodium). Despite some disagreement in the scientific community about the health benefits and risks associated with low-sodium diets,[16] most medical professionals agree that reducing the salt in our children's food is wise. The large majority of excess sodium in the average diet of an American child comes from processed food. So, eating meals that were cooked at home, using mostly fresh ingredients, can make a big difference to a child's salt and sodium intake. Attempting to eliminate salt entirely from a child's diet may not be the best way to go, either. Besides our biological need for small amounts of salt in our diets, salt can be used to flavor real, nutritious foods that support good health, thereby teaching our children a love of healthy foods.

Historically, salt has been a part of every world cuisine (traditionally added only in moderation) and culturally, it has been used as a symbol for flavor, good fortune, and happiness. In many communities, salt and bread is given to newlyweds to symbolize the family's wishes that the young couple should never go hungry and that their shared meals be flavorful. Beyond flavoring food, salt was used to cure meats and even heal wounds, because if its antiseptic properties. At certain points in history, salt was so valuable that soldiers were partially paid in salt. (This is the origin of the word "salary" and many common phrases like describing a competent person as being "worth his salt.")

PICKY EATERS AND FOOD PREFERENCES

Understanding the components of a balanced meal is an important concept for anyone trying to raise a healthy child. However, getting children to eat the foods provided for them can be an entirely separate challenge for a parent to overcome.

Especially in the developed world, where both food marketing to children and choices are excessive, many parents say they struggle to get their children to eat to healthful, real foods. The term "picky eater" is used commonly among parents, especially in countries where processed food consumption is high.

There are several formal and informal theories about why children refuse certain foods. There is evidence suggesting that age, tactile aversions to certain foods, eating environment, and the culture in which a child grows up can all influence a child's acceptance or rejection of foods.[17] In societies where processed foods dominate the diet, children may not be exposed to a wide enough variety of foods as babies and young children, so they resist new or unfamiliar foods later on. Some children may have a heightened sensitivity to the flavors and textures of certain foods, leading to true sensory aversions. It has also been suggested that children, having varying nutrient needs at different stages of growth, may crave a certain type of food and reject another during those periods. Certainly, there are very few parents in the world who would deliberately try to make their child a picky eater. So, supporting parents (and their children) through these phases is an important task for pediatricians, teachers, and anyone who helps to care for a child. Maintaining a stress-free environment during meals may be one of the biggest challenges for parents who are dealing with a picky eater but, as much as possible, meal times should be free of anxiety for the benefit of both parties. Perhaps the most powerful and often overlooked treatment for the picky eater syndrome is role modeling on the part of the parents. When parents consistently model enjoyment of healthful, diverse foods, children will often follow their lead. As with parenting in general, actions tend to speak louder than words.

Parent Forum

"Beeting" The Picky Eater Blues

My children will not eat beets ... or turnips, butternut squash, radishes, or sweet potatoes. And eggplant is absolutely out of the question. I probably have no right to complain. As kids go, they're good little eaters. They usually try at least some of the vegetables I cook and serve at dinner, but for some reason, the beet thing bothers me. I think it's because I really love beets and I want my children to share that love. You might think I'm crazy, but there are a few months of the year when I see those big red and gold bulbs stacked high at the farmers' market and I can practically taste the crunch of a raw shredded beet salad with fresh herbs and a tangy vinaigrette. My problem—the one I share with almost every parent I meet—is that no matter how hard I try, there are some foods my kids simply refuse to taste. Refuse. Period. It's frustrating, especially when I've tried to cook a delicious vegetable dish for dinner and it's met with cries of: "No way. Never in a million years," or "That looks gross, Mom!" After three children and ten years of parenting, I've been through my share of picky-eater phases. I remember a certain four-year-old who wanted to live on vanilla yogurt and another who begged for pasta with butter and parmesan—at every meal. I wish I'd known at the time that those phases would pass. I would have slept better at night and not felt like such a failure. The key, I've come to realize, is that I never gave up on the healthful foods I chose to eat when I was with them. Our actions speak far louder than our words at the dinner table! In fact, it was only when I stopped trying to get the kids to taste a bite of salad that our oldest son actually asked for some. I almost fell off my chair. He was watching his dad dive into a plate of crunchy greens and he suddenly decided that he wanted to be one of us! The best part: his younger brothers soon followed suit.

I think it's safe to say that the foods parents regularly eat at home will end up influencing the choices their children make. If our dinnertimes are usually colorful, nutritious occasions (and if fresh fruits and vegetables are regular features on the table), our kids will probably follow our lead ... eventually! So, if you've got a case of the picky-eater blues, here are a few simple tips that might help brighten your day.

1. Make sure you eat right. Enjoy fresh fruits and veggies IN FRONT of your kids, even if they don't want any.

2. Take your kids shopping for vegetables at the grocery store or, better yet, at the farmers' market. Let them see your excitement! It can be contagious.

3. Cook with your kids. Involve them in simple tasks that they can handle. (Even four-year-olds can chop mushrooms with a plastic knife or mash avocados in a bowl!)

4. When you eat out, hide the kids' menu. The sooner your kids eat the same foods you enjoy, the more fun you can have with them!

5. Try not to let picky eaters stress you out. I know it's hard, but anxiety at the dinner table tends to ruin everyone's meal. A wise woman once wrote: it's our job to provide children with a variety of healthy choices and it's their job to choose which of those foods (and how much) to eat.

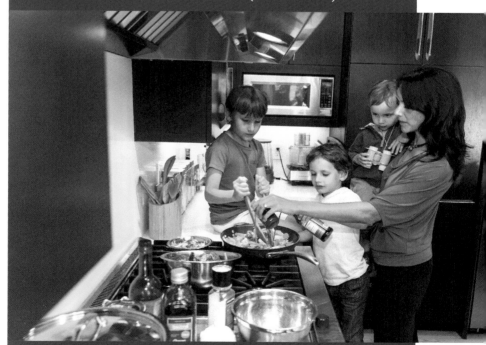

Figure 4.8   Cooking with children is a good way to encourage them to enjoy a variety of healthy foods.

CHAPTER 5

TASTE TRAINING: HOW FRENCH KIDS LEARN TO "GET TO YUM"

BY KAREN LE BILLON

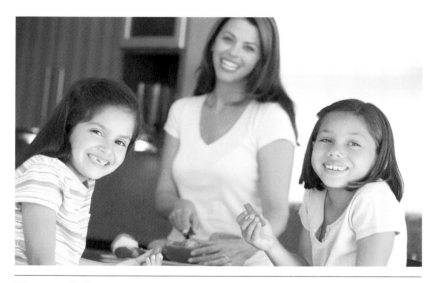

Figure 5.1

Children in France are educated to enjoy eating well: "French food education"
exposes them to a variety of real foods and flavors in the lunchroom as well as
the classroom. Many of these techniques can be tried at home, as mother and
professor Karen Le Billon found out when she moved with her French husband

and two young children to a small village in rural France. She posts examples of delicious French school lunches regularly on www.frenchkidseateverything.com, and her simple recipes, tips, and Taste Training plans are available on www.gettingtoyum.com.

Food education in France starts very young: as soon as Baby encounters solid food. Recommended first foods for babies include leek soup and endive. The top-selling cookbook on cooking for French babies includes vegetables like artichoke, celery, and cauliflower. Parents are encouraged to try dishes like sea bass with fennel ("why not serve it for your child's first birthday meal?") and—for the adventurous toddler—scallop tartare (yes, this means raw seafood—topped with minced pickles, capers, and white pepper, no less!).

By the time they start school (at age 3), French children have been exposed to a wider range of flavors than have German or English children. So it's perhaps unsurprising that dishes like radish salad, baked fish, roast

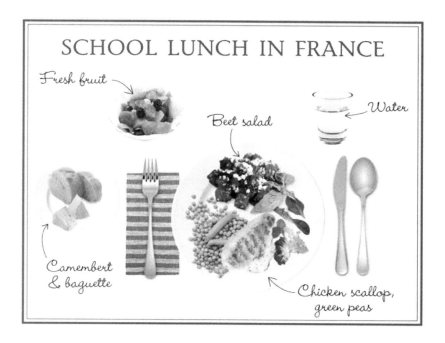

Figure 5.2   Typical School Lunch in France

guinea fowl, and cauliflower casserole regularly show up on their school lunch menus. As astounding as it may seem, most French kids actually eat all of this stuff. The reason is simple: they've learned to like it. In fact, they've been *taught* to like it—by parents and extended families, friends and peers, and teachers.

The French believe that teaching children to eat is a lot like teaching them to read. Now, *teaching* a child to eat might sound odd, because we often assume that kids' tastes are innate. How often have you heard a parent say about a child: "she (or he) is just a picky eater"? Although it's true that kids have different sensitivity levels for taste, their food *preferences* are learned—and are more nurture than nature. We don't often think of eating as something that you *learn*; more often than not, we assume that eating is just something that we *do*. But kids can learn to eat, just like they learn math or learn to read. Remember: it takes a long time to learn to read on your own, or to start doing advanced math! It's a process that takes years. But it is worth it: scientists have shown that exposing children to variety early on helps them to learn to like healthier foods for life. Moreover, the greater the variety of foods offered in the first two years of life, the more likely a child will be to eat healthily later on—even into adulthood.[1-3] And this really matters: early exposure to healthful foods is an important contributor to preventing obesity.[4]

The two main methods used to teach French children to enjoy eating healthy foods are lunchroom menus and in-class **Taste Training**. The menus are prepared in purpose-built kitchens and served in *cantines* (cafeterias) at all schools in France, following Ministry of Education regulations. These comprehensive regulations follow the dictum that "learning doesn't stop in the lunchroom," and treat eating as a pedagogical moment to be savored. **Health** is an important consideration: fried food is served no more than once per month, children drink only water at lunch, ketchup is only served with a small number of dishes, traditional cheeses or yogurts are served instead of flavored milk, portion sizes are limited (only one piece of baguette each!), and fresh fruit is served for dessert most days. But **variety** is equally important: the same dish can't be served more than once per month. Sound too much for your child to handle? Well, in France they can't opt out. Vending machines are banned in schools, and children can't bring lunches from home (unless they have an underlying medical issue).

Perhaps most important of all, the lunchroom menus are reinforced by Taste Training, in which children participate in a series of classroom-based games and lessons that teach them to understand the basic science of taste.

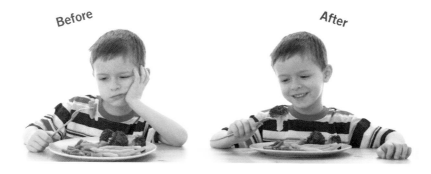

Figure 5.3   Through Taste Training, children learn to try new foods and improve their eating habits.

Children love the Taste Training activities, which include blindfold taste tests (first administered to the teacher, a guaranteed ice breaker); sampling the five tastes (salty, sweet, sour, bitter, and umami); and a "surprise sack" game in which guessing mystery foods underscores the link between texture and taste. As they grow older, more complex experiments, based on neurobiology and social psychology, are introduced. Children learn to "tame" their fears about new foods, and learn an important skill: how to be a competent eater and a (relatively) fearless taster of new foods.

Scientific studies have documented the significant effects of Taste Training, which improves children's eating habits and makes them more willing to try new foods.[2,3,5-11] In fact, scientific studies—in a diverse set of countries, including Finland, Korea, Britain, France, and the United States—show that Taste Training works better than traditional nutritionally based education methods.[12] That's why my second book, *Getting to Yum*, spells out the simple steps, recipes, and fun games that parents, teachers, and caregivers of all ages can use to try this method at home or at school. Good luck and happy eating!

Parent Forum

A Little Love in the Lunchbox
by Maya Adam

Among my most vivid childhood memories are the brown bag lunches my mother used to pack and send to school with us each day. Sometimes they had our names scribbled on the outside in black pen with a goofy smiley face. On Valentine's Day or my birthday, there would be a hastily written note and a small treat. My mother worked full time and raised two children without much help but she always managed to send a little love in our school lunches.

The foods in those lunches were simple: some reheated leftovers from the night before, packed in a thermos with a plastic spoon taped to the rim. There was always a piece of fruit, precut or pre-peeled so we could eat it easily, without too much mess. Sometimes, when she had baked cookies for us over the weekend, there would be something sweet in those bags, but usually the familiar smells of home were enough of a treat. Attending a school that didn't offer a hot lunch program, those lunches offered plenty of comfort in the middle of a long school day.

I was reminded of those brown bags of goodness a few weeks ago as I read an article suggesting that modern home-packed lunches are likely to be less nourishing than the meals offered in schools that meet new nutrition guidelines for the National School Lunch Program. (We're not yet playing in the same ballpark as the French school lunch program, but Michelle Obama certainly has been trying to get us closer!) The author of the article I read cited research studies that analyzed typical contents of home-packed lunches in two US states and compared them with what was being offered at school. Sadly, some of the most commonly packed items in today's "homemade lunch" were chips, sweetened drinks, and processed meats with highly refined crackers in the pre-packaged, disposable lunch containers sold at many supermarkets. When I picture that lunch, it's not hard to see how the brown bag has gotten such a bad rap. Clearly, the parents of today need convenient lunch solutions for their kids, but the truth is that packing a healthy home-cooked lunch isn't all that complicated. For parents who prefer to send lunch from home, here are a few practical tips:

1. Love your leftovers: Instead of tossing out that last serving of spaghetti Bolognese, reheat and pack it for lunch the next day. (Preheat your

child's thermos by rinsing it with boiling water to keep the contents hot until it's time to eat.)

2. Add some color: Veggies like carrots and cucumbers can be cut up the night before and stored in a zipper bag. With a small container of hummus or dip and a cool pack, your kids can enjoy a tangy, crunchy side dish.

3. Think like a kid: Cut up or peel fruits and pack them in small containers or zipper bags. This makes them more manageable for small hands and mouths. As lunch periods get shorter, ready-to-eat fruits can also save time for kids.

I'm a big fan of the recent school lunch reforms—and happy to know that my children would be well fed if I didn't send them lunches from home. But as long as I can swing it (and as long as they keep asking me to) I'll pack their lunches with foods that provide more than just nutrients. I'll fill their bags with a little bit of love.

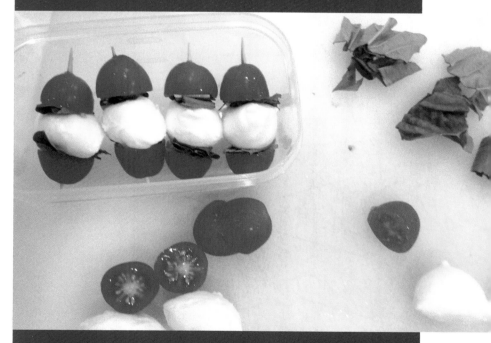

Figure 5.4 Packing a healthy lunch is easier than many parents think.

CHAPTER 6

THE CASE FOR FAMILY DINNER

BY JENNY ROSENSTRACH

Over the past five years, I've written over 750 posts about family dinner for my blog Dinner: A Love Story. Out of that blog came two books about dinner—a collection of recipes, strategies, and tons of tips and tricks for how to feed hungry, growing, often picky kids. What qualified me to do all this? Get a load of this credential: With the help of my husband, I cook dinner every night for our family of four. Always have, always will. Yep. Today that seems to be unusual enough to be a major qualification, because people ask me all the time: How do you find the time to do it? How do you figure out what to make that everyone will like, including kids? How do you have family dinner and not lose your mind?

When I was growing up, it wasn't even called family dinner. It was called dinner—the "family" part was a given. Somewhere between then and now, we all got busy. We got used to the convenience of takeout and prepared foods. We signed our kids up for activities that cut right into dinner hour. The economy got tough and we had to take two jobs or shifts that weren't necessarily conducive to roasting a chicken. We became used to the idea that since the office can reach us 24/7, we should in fact be *available* 24/7. There are all kinds of legitimate reasons eating with our kids isn't a priority anymore—I'm not here to judge anyone and the choices they make. I know that for every parent who manages to squeeze in some quality bonding time over the lasagna, there's another parent who figures out how to do it at the breakfast table or in the car or on the

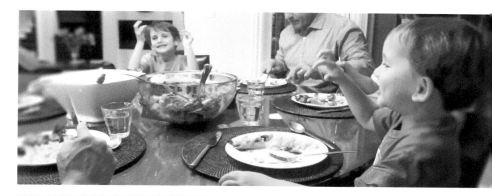

Figure 6.1   Dinner: a ritual that can bring families together on a daily basis.

chairlift. But if you are in search of a ritual that will bring the family together, a ritual that will satisfy a deep craving to find meaning in the everyday, family dinner is where it's at. At least it always has been for me.

Why do I depend on it so much? I've written about the trickle-down theory of family dinner, which goes like this: When you prioritize eating well, there is a good chance that a lot of other things naturally fall into place. Such as:

You'll work more efficiently: It was the musician Jack White who said "Deadlines are your friends, they are productivity gods." I quote this because if you think of dinner as the deadline at the end of every workday—"I have to get home to make that chicken by 6:30"—I can guarantee you will get more done at the office in order to make that happen.

You'll spend less money: If you get in the habit of doing a weekly shop, you'll have options when you get home from work and will be less likely to fall back on takeout or processed foods from the freezer.

You know what's going into your kids' bodies (at least once a day): When you make your own food, you know exactly what's going into that food. It's un- realistic for most people to make everything from scratch every single day—*we* certainly don't, um, hello Trader Joe's hash browns!—but if you set the bar that high, you're more likely to hit a level you're comfortable with.

You'll have built-in bonding time: I don't know about you, but I can spend a whole day with my kids—driving them all over, nagging them about hanging up their jackets or taking a shower, or signing their eight zillion hand-outs—and not have a single meaningful interaction with them. Knowing we'll all be eyeball-to-eyeball at 7:30, no phones, no interruptions, no handouts, makes such a difference in my overall outlook of *every single day*. Keep the ritual up long enough and your kids will view the table less as a place to consume the pork chops and more as a safe place to talk about anything. Or maybe nothing. You can't always force the connecting, but I will say that it's nice to have a system in place that is *conducive* for connecting.

Maybe I'm preaching to the converted here. Maybe you want to make family dinner happen, but you don't know *how* to make family dinner happen? Well, let's just say, you are definitely not alone. I have a couple tips and tricks that can help get you started.

Find Your Rotation: Just because the food is secondary to the main event (sitting down together) doesn't mean the food is not important. Good food is the draw and having a rotation of easy meals is crucial to the equation for everyone involved. If you're in need of suggestions you'll find a few of my favorite recipes at the end of this chapter. The most important thing you're looking for in a weeknight recipe is simplicity. If you are breaking out ten pots and pans and tracking down exotic ingredients, I am here to tell you that you will be about one thousand times less likely to cook again the next night.

Make a Plan and Shop for the Week: Again, if you have a plan, you're much less likely to succumb to the siren call of takeout or freezer food. Take a minute to think about what's for dinner before you leave for work in the morning and get your head around what has to happen when you walk in the door first thing—chop an onion, boil a pot of water? Get the momentum going as soon as you can, even if it's the morning. Your post-work self will be so appreciative that your pre-work self thought to make a vinaigrette for the salad.

Kids Don't Like What You Like? Try Deconstructing Dinner: This has become more than a strategy at our dinner table—it's now a philosophy. I can look at almost any meal that's potentially offensive to my kids and break it down into parts that are actually appealing to them. The key to this, obviously, is to make sure a few of those parts are foods that your kids are not just going to put up with eating, but foods that they're also excited about eating. So in other words, you might want to come at dinner ideas backward. For instance, let's say your kid is a pasta junkie—that he spends every waking moment wondering who he has to rob in order to eat it again. Instead of wishing he would just try something else, build on his love for pasta. Consider making Pasta with Roast Butternut Squash (see recipe below). If he doesn't eat the squash, at least he'll have that positive outlook when he sits down at the table. That's what you're going for. I find that the longer I can keep my kids' minds open, the better chance I have of getting them to try new foods.

Commit: I can give you all the recipes in the world; I can share my mental archive of time-saving, money-saving, sanity-saving kitchen tips; I can give you pep talks until you want to suffocate me with my pom-poms; but without the conviction to make it happen, it won't be possible. There is no magic button. Family dinner requires front-end planning, plus lots of back-end chopping and mincing and assembling. Once you realize that it's going to be a little work, once you embrace that work, your head will be in a much better place. And you will be happy to be there.

PASTA WITH ROAST BUTTERNUT SQUASH

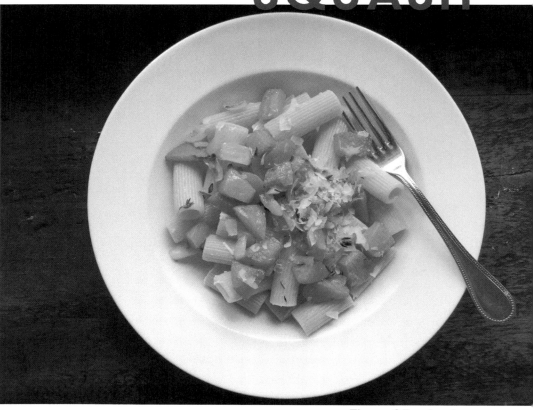

Time: 35 minutes

INGREDIENTS

3 cups (about 24 ounces) chopped butternut squash (or 1 large squash that has been peeled, seeded, and chopped; but I implore you: buy it already chopped)

½ onion, chopped

leaves from 4 or 5 fresh thyme sprigs

3 tablespoons olive oil salt and pepper to taste

2 teaspoons smoked paprika

1 pound any pasta (I like pappardelle or penne)

½ cup freshly grated Parmesan, plus more for serving

fresh ricotta (optional), for serving

DIRECTIONS

1. Preheat the oven to 425°F.

2. In a baking dish lined with foil, toss together the squash, onions, thyme, olive oil, salt and pepper, and paprika. Roast for about 30 minutes, or until the squash is brown around the edges and is tender when pierced with a fork.

3. Meanwhile, prepare the pasta according to the package directions, reserving ¼ cup of pasta water before draining.

4. Return the drained pasta to the pot and toss with the squash.

5. Add the Parmesan with half of the reserved pasta water to thin and evenly distribute the cheese. Add the remaining pasta water if needed. Serve topped with more Parmesan and ricotta if desired.

MAPLE CANDY PORK CHOPS

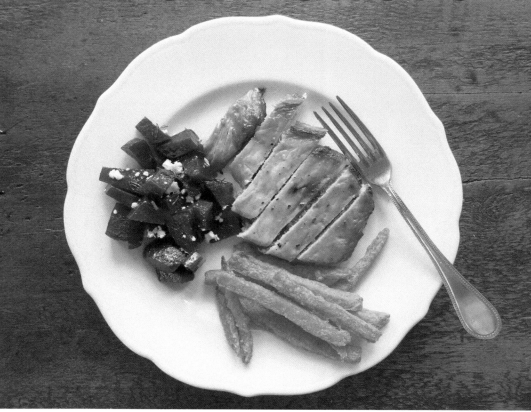

Time: 25 minutes (plus an hour's marinating time)

INGREDIENTS

4 boneless center-cut pork chops

⅓ cup pure maple syrup

3 tablespoons canola oil

¼ cup low-sodium soy sauce

¼ cup rice wine vinegar

1 garlic clove, halved, or a shake or two of powdered garlic

DIRECTIONS

1. Place the pork chops in a zipper bag. Add the maple syrup, canola oil, soy sauce, rice wine vinegar, and garlic. Marinate anywhere from 60 minutes to overnight.

2. When ready to cook, preheat the oven to 450°F. Remove the chops from the marinade and pat dry with paper towels, scraping off any garlic that clings to the meat. Place the chops on a foil-lined rimmed baking sheet and bake for 15 to 20 minutes, flipping once halfway through, until firm in the center but not rock hard.

FRIED CHICKPEAS WITH YOGURT SAUCE AND NAAN

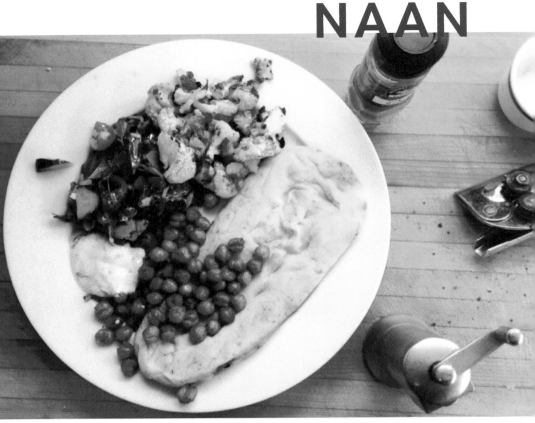

INGREDIENTS

oil for frying

2 14-ounce cans of garbanzo beans

salt, pepper and cayenne to taste

½ teaspoon garlic salt

½ teaspoon paprika

¾ cup plain yogurt

1 teaspoon garam masala

squeeze of lime juice

1 tablespoon olive oil

chopped cilantro and mint

naan to serve

DIRECTIONS

1. Add a generous amount of oil to a cast iron skillet set over medium-high heat. Drain, rinse, and dry two 14-ounce cans of garbanzo beans. When pan is hot but not smoking, add beans (in batches, if necessary, or two pans—you want a single layer of beans on the pan's surface). Fry about 15 minutes, tossing every 5 minutes or so. Remove with a slotted spoon into a paper-towel-lined bowl. Once all chickpeas are fried and drained, add salt, pepper, a pinch of cayenne, and a ½ teaspoon of both garlic salt and paprika.

2. While the chickpeas fry, whisk together about ¾ cup plain yogurt with a teaspoon garam masala, squeeze of lime juice, tablespoon or so of olive oil, and chopped cilantro and/or mint. Salt and pepper to taste.

3. Toast naan and serve with yogurt sauce and chickpeas.

BLACK BEAN AND GOAT CHEESE QUESADILLAS

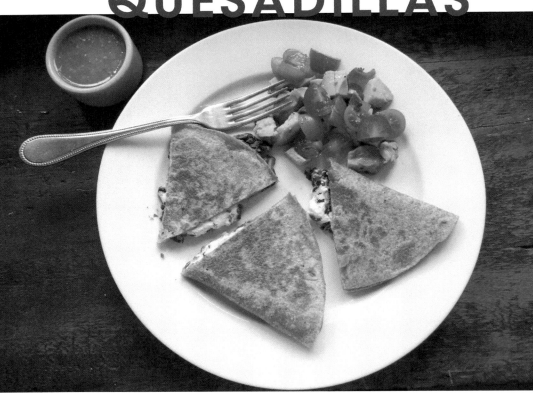

Time: 25 minutes

INGREDIENTS

2 tablespoons vegetable oil

2 garlic cloves, finely chopped

1 teaspoon ground cumin

2 15-ounce cans black beans, rinsed and drained

salt and pepper to taste

3 scallions (white and light green parts only), chopped

5 8-inch whole-wheat tortillas

5 ounces goat cheese

salsa or salsa verde, for dipping

DIRECTIONS

1. In a large skillet, heat the oil over medium heat. Add the garlic and cumin and stir until the garlic is golden, about 1 minute. Stir in the beans, salt, and pepper, mashing everything with a large fork. Add 1/3 cup water and the scallions and cook, stirring until most of the water is absorbed, 2 to 3 minutes. Remove from the heat.

2. Set a separate skillet over medium-high heat and add a shot of cooking spray. Place one tortilla in the skillet, spreading about a fifth of the bean filling on one side. Sprinkle a fifth of the goat cheese on top of the beans and fold the other half of the tortilla over to seal. Flip around a few times until the tortilla is golden on both sides and the cheese is melted, 2 to 3 minutes. Remove to a dinner plate and tent with foil to keep warm. Repeat with the remaining tortillas. Cut each into three or four wedges and serve with salsa or salsa verde.

Parent Forum

Little Celebrations
By Maya Adam

A very smart friend once told me that happiness is simply a mathematical ratio of reality over expectations. The less realistic our expectations, the less chance we'll have of being satisfied with the end product. I think this is a valuable formula to keep in mind when we're cooking. If we aim for absolute perfection when we cook, it's less likely that we'll be able to over-look the little flaws and enjoy the goodness in our homemade dishes. If the pancakes aren't completely round, they can still taste delicious! More importantly, they're made with love and sometimes the real goodness is on the inside!

Could it be that one of the reasons the average American adult spends only 27 minutes in the kitchen each day is that we're afraid of failing? What if we modified our expectations so that all we're aiming for is real food combined in ways that we think our families might enjoy?

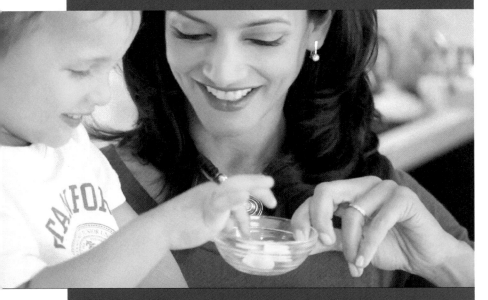

Figure 6.6 Successful home cooking involves experimenting with simple ingredients, combined in ways we think we will enjoy.

The high-wire kind of cooking we sometimes see on television shows is impressive, no question. But for most of us, trying to do that every night is like trying to reenact a Cirque du Soleil production at home, after a long and busy day. I'm not suggesting we shouldn't stretch ourselves at times by trying to make things we once thought were beyond our abilities in the kitchen, but the more forgiving we are of slightly overcooked fish or slightly under-salted pasta, the more likely it will be that our pots find their way out of the cupboard for an encore. Funny enough, cooking (and eating) together with the people we love has the potential to influence our happiness calculations as well. Cooking and eating together, whenever we can, is one way to optimize the "reality" part of the equation. By seeing our meals as a way of honoring the moment, our family dinners not only help us to eat more healthfully, but they can also remind us to celebrate each day, one meal at a time. There's no need to put on a performance with every prop in place before the curtain rises. If we aim to be real instead of being perfect when we cook, we can turn ordinary days into little celebrations and happiness will be on the menu every day of the week.

CHAPTER 7

FOOD MARKETING TO CHILDREN

BY JESSICA ALMY[i]

SENIOR NUTRITION POLICY COUNSEL AT THE
CENTER FOR SCIENCE IN THE
PUBLIC INTEREST.

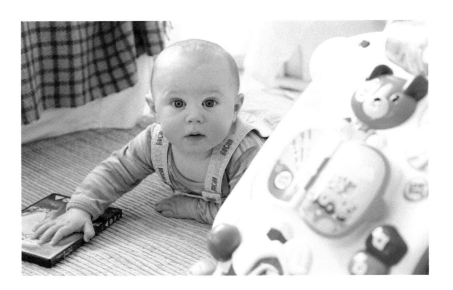

Figure 7.1 Brand affinities are set early in life.

---

[i] The author would like to thank Dr. Margo G. Wootan, nutrition policy director, for her insight and guidance.

WHY FOOD MARKETING MATTERS

Food marketing affects children's food preferences, food choices, and their health. Toddlers can recognize brands in the store before they are able to read. Kindergarteners can typically name a brand of soda, third-graders can name two brands, and sixth-graders can name three.

Children are inundated with food marketing every day. Marketing to children is big business: food companies in the US spend approximately $1.8 billion each year on it. Why? Children spend $25 billion on purchases and influence another $200 billion in household purchases each year. Moreover, brand affinities—preferences for one brand of cola over another, for example—are set early in life.

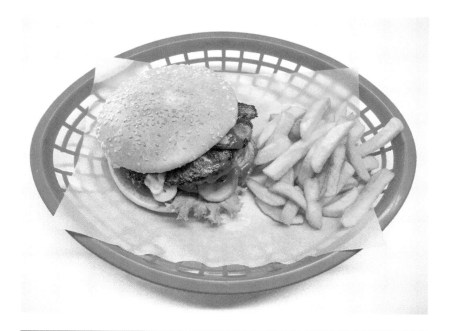

Figure 7.2.1 The majority of advertisements targeted towards kids are for unhealthy foods and sugary drinks.

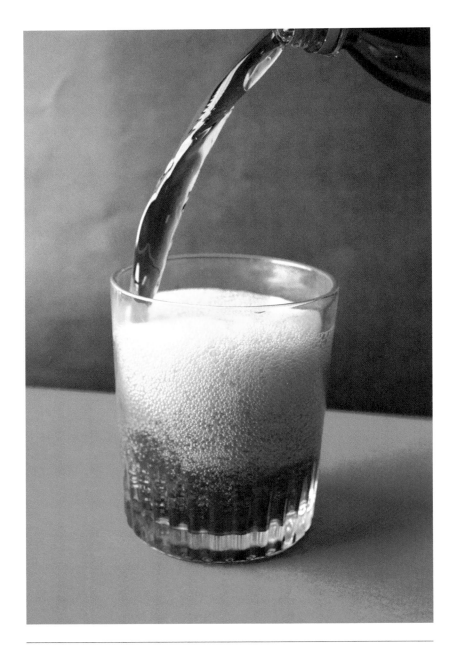

Figure 7.2.2

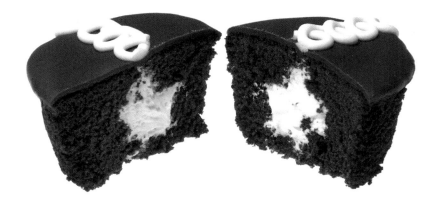

Figure 7.2.3

The American Psychological Association concluded that until the age of about eight years, children are unable to understand the persuasive intent of advertisements. More recent research reveals that some children as old as 11 or 12 may not understand advertisements' persuasive intent. However, even children who do recognize that marketing is designed to sell them something are not protected from its effects. Companies know that marketing works or they would not spend so much money on it.

If food companies were in the business of advertising and marketing mostly fruits, vegetables, and whole grains to children, food marketing would not be a problem. The problem is that the overwhelming majority of foods marketed to children are of poor nutritional value. In a recent study, three out of every four food advertisements on the popular children's television network Nickelodeon were for unhealthy foods. Also, restaurant children's menus are dominated by unhealthy foods and beverages. Children eat too many sugary, salty foods made from refined grains, and a third of children are overweight or obese. They do not need further inducement to eat unhealthy foods or drink soda and other sugary drinks.

Foods marketed to children often have excessive quantities of salt, sugars, or fat, which are added to extend the shelf life of food products, mask off-tastes that result from processing and storage, or make products harder to resist. In addition, almost all of the foods marketed to children lack the positive nutrition that fruits, vegetables, and whole grains provide. In fact, some of the least healthy foods are made for and marketed specifically to children. Cereal manufacturers, for example, advertise their healthiest products to adults and their least healthy varieties to children.

In the United States, food marketing to children has been left primarily to self-regulation. There are few laws limiting advertising to children. The

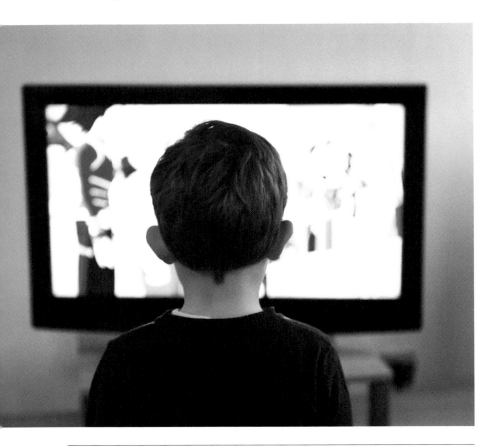

Figure 7.3 Despite efforts to curb marketing to children, children may be exposed to 10-15 commercials in a single thirty minute show.

Children's Television Act, passed in 1990, limits the quantity of advertising during children's television programming to 10.5 minutes of advertising during every hour of children's programming on the weekends and 12 minutes each hour during the week. Given that commercials run in 15- or 30-second slots, it is not uncommon for children to be exposed to ten or fifteen commercials during a single half-hour show. In addition, although television advertising remains a major way that companies market to children, companies use a wide array of approaches to promote unhealthy food to kids.

FORMS OF FOOD MARKETING TO CHILDREN

When most people think of marketing, they picture television, magazine, and Internet advertising, which are forms of *promotion*. When it comes to food, however, advertising is only one kind of marketing. In addition, food companies use images, claims, and design on packaging and add fat, sugar, and salt, colors, shapes, or other appealing qualities to make the *product* more enticing to customers. Retailers and manufacturers employ low *prices* and sales to encourage purchases. And working together, food manufacturers and retailers also use the *placement* of products at eye level, in places in high-traffic areas, such as the end of aisles or the checkout, to generate sales. These four techniques—promotion, product, price, and placement—are the "4 Ps" of marketing.

Promotion is a significant marketing approach that encompasses advertisements during children's television programming, in children's magazines, and on websites and apps. Nearly half of the money that food companies spend on marketing to children is spent on these kinds of promotions, although the media mix is shifting. From 2006 to 2009, food companies' spending on new media—which includes online, mobile, and viral marketing to kids—increased by 50 percent.

Promotions are not limited to screens, however. In restaurants, promotions can take the form of the toys that are included with children's meals. Children may order the meal because they want the toy, rather than because of any inherent quality of the food.

Food companies also spend $149 million each year on in-school marketing. This money goes toward getting food company logos and brand names on books, school supplies, school signs, scoreboards, sports equipment, and posters, as well as on vending machines and display racks in school cafeterias. In Montgomery County, Maryland, for example, about 80 percent of schools had posters or signs with food and beverage marketing, most of which was for restaurants, prepared foods, and soda.

Additionally, the $149 million a year that food companies spend on in-school marketing does not include the (free) labor of the parents, educators, and children who are enlisted to participate in school marketing schemes. Sunny Delight, for example, produces fruit-flavored sugar drinks. Through a program called Book Spree, Sunny Delight provides books to schools in exchange for proofs of purchase (labels) from its products. What is positioned by the company as a charitable endeavor is actually a clever marketing ploy that requires schools to encourage families to buy unhealthy beverages and have children ferry labels to school. In this way, Sunny Delight gets valuable word-of-mouth advertising in exchange for its "donations" to schools.

The product itself is a core approach to marketing. First, there is the composition of the product. For example, by selling crackers, meat, cheese, candy, and a drink as a single product, Kraft makes its Lunchables products more desirable to busy parents as a convenient all-in-one meal solution. Lunchables also appeal to children as something they can assemble themselves. Lunchables have become an entire supermarket category. Fruit snacks are another example. By shaping sugar, wax or gelatin, colors and dyes, and sometimes a bit of fruit juice or fruit puree into the form of Spiderman or Hello Kitty, food companies have created a new category of food that they market to parents as a healthy snack. Thus, candy is positioned as "fruit" and has become a regular addition to lunchboxes.

Second, package designs often use characters, colors, and shapes designed to appeal to children. Companies use colors like red to signal sweetness and excitement, employ cartoonish script or crayoned fonts, or include child-oriented puzzles, games, and contests to appeal to kids. In addition, companies use licensed characters like SpongeBob SquarePants and use their own "spokescharacters," such as the General Mills Trix Rabbit on packaging.

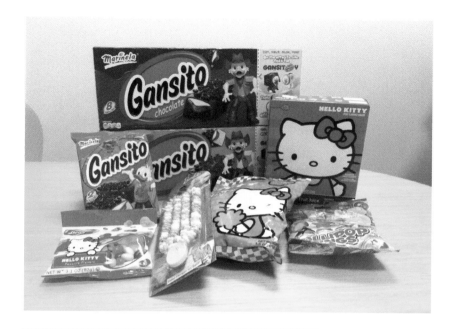

Figure 7.4   Bright colors and popular media characters are often used to make packaged foods more appealing to children.

Likewise, restaurants market foods to children by promoting them on children's menus, which are typically less expensive than other meals on the menu. Unfortunately, the vast majority of children's meals at chain restaurants are unhealthful. In fact, more than half of the top chain restaurants do not offer a single healthy option on the children's menu. The default beverages and side dishes—that is, the drinks and sides customers get if they do not request another—are usually unhealthy options like fries and soda.

Finally, there is placement. Placement may be the most subtle form of food marketing, but it is also one of the most pervasive and effective. Retail analyst Herb Sorensen contends that the "most important promotion is place, not price" in the grocery industry. Because the average supermarket stocks 30,000 to 50,000 items and people typically buy 300 to 400 different products each year, people are unable to pay attention to the vast majority of the products in the store. Thus, food companies pay extra money to have their products placed where they will get the most attention on supermarket shelves.

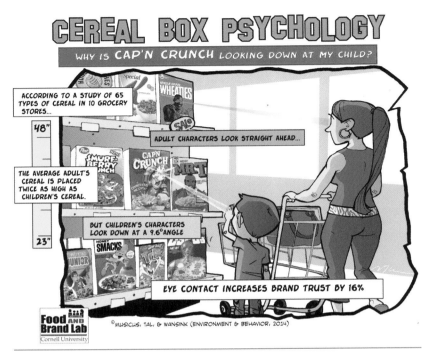

Figure 7.5   Aviva Musicus, Aner Tal, and Brian Wansink (2014). Eyes in the Aisles: Why is Cap'n Crunch Looking Down at My Child? Environment & Behavior. DOI: 10.1177/0013916514528793

Commonly used placement techniques include the amount of space allocated to a particular food product and the use of high-visibility areas, such as the middle of a shelf or end of an aisle. Supermarkets use placement to market particular foods to children by putting child-oriented products at their eye level or within reach.

Together, these four marketing techniques—promotion, product, price, and placement—influence the foods and beverages that children request, what they buy with their own money, and what they eat.

PROTECTING CHILDREN FROM FOOD MARKETING

Parents and food companies have a shared responsibility to protect the health of children. Although parents' understanding of marketing and nutrition can help them make good choices for their children, these good choices become more difficult when families are inundated with food marketing. And, of course, children are not always in the care of their parents. Children are exposed to food marketing and make decisions about food in a wide variety of settings, including while they are in school, at friends' houses, and in the care of extended family.

In the modern food environment, making good nutritional choices takes a great deal of time and energy, because so many foods that appear to be healthy, or are explicitly marketed as such, are not. In one study, researchers examined the nutritional quality of foods directed to children in a Canadian supermarket. Excluding candy, soda and other sugary drinks, cakes, and potato chips—which most parents know are unhealthy—the researchers still found that 89 percent of the food products marketed to children were of "poor nutritional quality," primarily because they contained too much salt, sugar, or fat. Among the unhealthy products were breakfast cereal, crackers, fruit snacks, granola bars, pasta, frozen waffles, cheese, and yogurt drinks.

Two approaches can protect children from unhealthy food marketing: the industry can adopt voluntary measures to reduce or eliminate unhealthy food marketing to children, or the government can regulate food marketing to children. For the most part, the United States and many other countries have relied primarily on a self-regulatory approach.

SELF-REGULATION

Under self-regulation, an industry sets and enforces guidelines itself. Effective self-regulation can ward off government interventions and can ensure that the most progressive companies—the good actors—do not suffer competitive harm by going above and beyond the bare minimum that the law requires. However, in many contexts (not only food marketing to children), self-regulation is criticized on principle as letting the fox guard the hen house. Additionally, some companies may not participate in voluntary self-regulation or self-regulatory guidelines may be weak.

In the United States, the Council of Better Business Bureaus administers two self-regulatory programs regarding food marketing to children. One, the Children's Advertising Review Unit (CARU), provides guidelines to define misleading and inaccurate advertisements and investigates complaints regarding misleading advertising to children (all advertising, not just ads for food). CARU's voluntary guidelines cover print, radio, television, and Internet advertising. The other, the Children's Food and Beverage Advertising Initiative (CFBAI), addresses the nutritional quality of the products marketed to children.

CFBAI sets nutrition criteria, which its member companies agree to apply to marketing as defined by the program. For example, the companies participating in CFBAI may only advertise to children cereals that have 10 grams of sugar or less per one-ounce serving size.

Critics of CFBAI point out that it defines marketing narrowly, not encompassing on-package marketing, toy premiums, or in-store marketing displays geared to children. Additionally, the program protects only children under age 12, and some of the foods permitted under the nutrition standards, such as Cocoa Puffs and Popsicles, are not foods that most nutrition experts consider healthful.

Internationally, some food companies participate in the International Food and Beverage Alliance or the EU Pledge, both of which limit some forms of food marketing to children. Neither program is significantly stronger than CFBAI. Both programs continue to allow marketing unhealthy foods to children by, for example, including toys in Happy Meals or putting Tony the Tiger on boxes of cereal.

In addition to the programs administered by the Council of Better Business Bureaus, in the United States, the National Restaurant Association has a restaurant certification program called Kids LiveWell. Created in July 2011, Kids LiveWell requires that member restaurants offer and highlight at least one meal and one side dish that meet the program's nutrition standards. Approximately 100 restaurants and chains participate.

However, like CFBAI, Kids LiveWell has significant limitations. The primary problem is that the program requires that only one meal and side dish on the children's menu meet nutrition standards. This gives parents and children

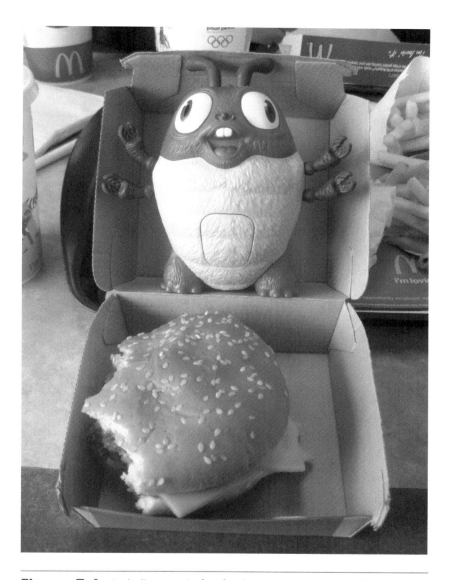

Figure 7.6 Including toys in fast food meals encourages children to eat unhealthy foods.

limited choices and means that most children's menus continue to be dominated by unhealthy options.

To date, the results from self-regulation are mixed. The good news is that seventeen companies, including some of the largest food companies in the United States, participate in CFBAI, covering about 80 percent of the food advertising during children's television programming. However, a number of companies that market to children do not participate in CFBAI and have not adopted any policies to limit marketing to children. Of 128 food manufacturers, chain restaurants, television stations, kids' magazines, and video gaming, toy, and other companies that market food to children, three-quarters of the companies either do not have a policy on food marketing to children or else their policy is very weak. Whereas nearly two-thirds of food and beverage manufacturers have marketing policies, only a quarter of restaurants and entertainment companies do.

A number of studies show that self-regulation is resulting in some decline in unhealthful food marketing to children. However, they also show that progress is slow and limited. On Nickelodeon, for example, ads that are for unhealthy foods declined from about 90 percent of all food advertisements before self-regulation was in place to 70 percent of the network's food advertisements now. Companies can and should do better.

Additionally, few media and entertainment companies are stepping up to take responsibility for their full range of marketing to children. Qubo was the first media company to remove unhealthy food marketing in its full range of media. Disney followed suit with a commitment to remove junk food ads on television, radio, and its websites by 2015. Disney also has changed the defaults for beverages to healthy choices, such as 100% juice, water, and low-fat milk, and offers fruits and vegetables as the default side dishes with children's meals in its theme parks. These changes have been well received; two-thirds of families stick with the healthy defaults for children's meals.

In summary, some companies have adopted voluntary policies to limit some of their advertising to children. However, many food, beverage, restaurant, and entertainment companies still market foods that are unhealthy to children. In addition, voluntary policies rarely cover marketing via in-school programs, branded fundraisers, children's menus and toy premiums in restaurants. Nearly all food manufacturers fail to address their marketing through child-oriented packages, and no food companies or retailers have food marketing policies that prohibit the placement of unhealthy foods at children's eye level, on endcaps, or at checkout.

GOVERNMENT POLICY

The World Health Organization has issued recommendations on the marketing of food and non-alcoholic beverages to children. Those recommendations state that governments should be the "key stakeholders in the development of policy" to protect children from harmful food marketing.

In the United States, the federal government has chosen to take a fairly passive role in limiting food marketing to children. Some government policies address deceptive advertising and invasions of privacy. The Federal Trade Commission (FTC) has the authority to prosecute deceptive advertisements and prohibit websites from collecting information from children under the age of 13 without parental consent. However, no government policy broadly applies nutrition standards to the foods that can be advertised or otherwise marketed to children.

This passive approach is a product of history. Twice, the federal government has attempted to take a more active role in protecting children from unhealthy food marketing. Each of these attempts, however, has been thwarted by significant industry pushback. In the 1970s, responding to a petition from public interest groups, FTC lawyers proposed a rule—dubbed "kidvid" by the media—that sought to ban television advertising (not just food ads) to very young children and provide some protections for older children. However, food, toy, and entertainment companies lobbied aggressively to prevent the proposed policies from taking effect.

Decades later, in 2009, Congress directed the FTC, together with the Food and Drug Administration, the Centers for Disease Control and Prevention, and the Department of Agriculture, to establish an Interagency Working Group (IWG) on Food Marketed to Children to develop a set of principles on food marketing to children. The principles were not intended to constitute binding policy or regulation, but rather to set voluntary model nutrition standards for food marketing to children and to clarify what communications constitute marketing directed to children. However, before the IWG could issue its final recommendations, it too was disbanded under intense industry lobbying.

Despite these setbacks, recent developments promise to offer some protection to children. In schools, new Smart Snacks regulations impose nutritional standards for the foods sold through vending machines, à la carte lines, school stores, and some fundraisers. And the Department of Agriculture has proposed a rule that would require that schools address the marketing of unhealthy foods and beverages on school campuses through their local wellness policies.

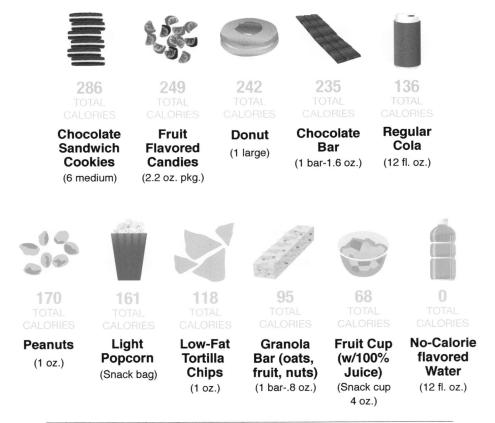

Figure 7.7 The Healthy Hunger Free Act of 2010 improved the quality of school snacks. The top and bottom rows reflect school snacks from before and after the new standards.

Further, some states and municipalities are working to limit unhealthful food marketing to children, especially where there are gaps in self-regulation. Because no restaurants apply their marketing standards to toy giveaways with children's meals—a common and popular form of marketing—Santa Clara County and San Francisco, for example, have passed laws to improve the nutritional quality and marketing of restaurant children's meals.

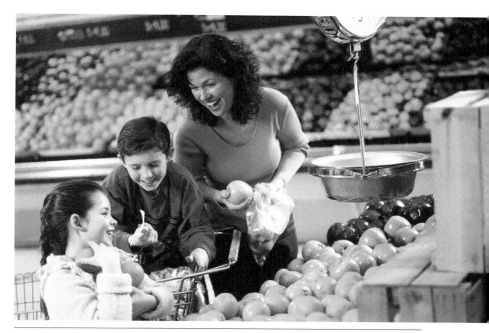

Figure 7.8   Parents can play an active role in limiting their children's exposure to marketing for unhealthful foods.

Globally, the governments of some countries have taken a more active role than the United States. Mexico, for example, prohibits advertisements for chocolate, candy, chips, and soda on children's television and movies, imposing a fine of approximately $75,000 for each violation of the law. Norway also limits broadcast advertisements to children.

Despite these developments, however, the problems posed by food marketing to children remain a public health concern. Keeping in mind the 4 Ps of marketing—promotion, product, price, and placement—you can see how efforts to limit advertising do not fully address all the ways that food marketing pervades children's lives and affects their diets and health.

Parents concerned about the effects of unhealthful food marketing on their children can ask food and beverage manufacturers, entertainment companies, and restaurants to do more, whether by joining self-regulatory programs or by expanding the scope of their policies to include all forms of marketing. Parents can also discuss their concerns about food marketing to children with their elected officials and support policy initiatives designed to protect children from food marketing.

CHAPTER 8

FOOD ALLERGIES, INTOLERANCES, AND CELIAC DISEASE

FOOD ALLERGIES

In most parts of the world, awareness about childhood food allergies has increased dramatically in recent decades. Recent reviews of the scientific literature on food allergies in Europe, Asia, and the United States estimate that 3% to 5% of adults and 3% to 8% of children are currently suffering from one or more food allergies.[1-4] This said, there is some disagreement about the magnitude of the true changes in prevalence in recent decades. Some studies have also suggested that perhaps increasing public awareness has led to a greater number of parents reporting food allergies in their children.[2] Regardless of the disagreement over the magnitude of the changing prevalence, researchers and medical professionals agree that the contemporary management of food allergies poses a very significant challenge for children and their families. Beyond the potentially serious adverse health consequences, food allergies can impact social interactions, school attendance, perceived quality of life, and even the financial security of the family. For these reasons, the successful management of food allergies should take on a holistic approach, addressing both medical and psychosocial concerns in an attempt to normalize and stabilize the day-to-day life of the child.

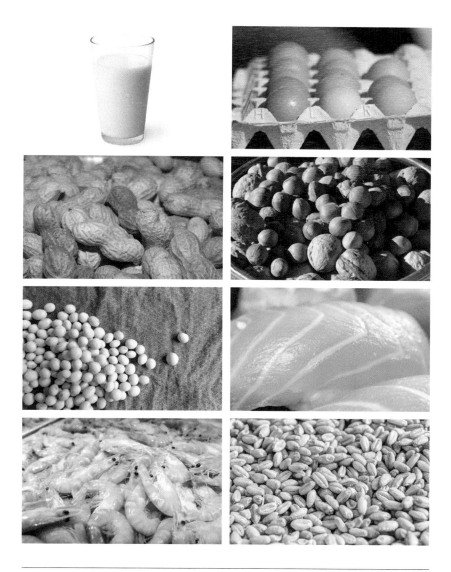

Figure 8.1.1– 8.1.8 The most common food allergens: milk, eggs, peanuts, tree nuts, soy, fish, shellfish and wheat.

Allergies to a wide variety of foods have been documented, but only a relatively small group of foods account for the majority of allergic reactions. The most common food allergens are in milk, eggs, peanuts, tree nuts, soy, fish, shellfish, and wheat. The allergic response to these food allergens is triggered by a specific component of that food, usually a protein that the body mistakenly recognizes as a threat. Reactions can range from mild to severe, including the potentially life-threatening reaction known as anaphylaxis. An anaphylactic reaction is actually a grossly exaggerated attempt on the part of the child's immune system to protect the child from the perceived threat. The dilation of blood vessels and narrowing of airways that often results from this kind of reaction can end up causing difficulty breathing and a precipitous drop in blood pressure. Both of these are potentially life threatening for an allergic child. Some of the early signs and symptoms of anaphylaxis are itching and swelling of the face, throat, and tongue, difficulty breathing, and the appearance of hives on the skin. Immune-mediated food allergies can also result in more chronic problems, including skin rashes and other non-life-threatening reactions.

WHAT CAUSED THE RISE IN FOOD ALLERGIES?

The increasing prevalence of food allergies, documented in many parts of the world, has spawned a great deal of scientific research focused on exploring the underlying causes of this trend. While there are no definitive answers as yet, several theories have been proposed. Some of these theories are summarized below.

1. One theory suggests that the Western diet has increased children's susceptibility to developing allergies by decreasing the biodiversity of bacteria normally residing in the gut. A study conducted by the National Academy of Sciences[5] compared the intestinal bacteria from children in Florence, Italy, with those of children living in a rural African village in Burkina Faso. Significant differences in the variety of intestinal flora were observed between these two groups. The African children who took part in the study lived in subsistence-farming

communities that produced their own food and consumed a mainly vegetarian diet. Within these communities, a significantly lower incidence of food allergies was documented. In contrast, the Italian children who took part in the study consumed a diet that was comparatively higher in animal fats, sugars, and other processed foods, and also had a higher incidence of food allergies. The study authors postulate that a Western diet may lead to less-diversified gut flora. They also suggest that exposing children to an array of microbes that are ingested with food may offer some protection against developing food allergies, by desensitizing the immune system to potential food allergens.

2. The hygiene hypothesis is another potential explanation for the rising rates of allergies and asthma diagnoses. This hypothesis suggests that due to dramatic improvements in cleaning methods and hygiene practices, children may actually be underexposed to the diverse array of microbes needed to facilitate proper development of the immune system. In support of this hypothesis, there is some evidence suggesting that people living on farms develop fewer allergies than those living in urban settings[6] and that the immune function of children growing up in rural environments may actually be enhanced by regular exposure to a wide variety of microbes.

3. Other researchers have examined the timing of exposure to common food allergens, like those in nuts and shellfish. Some of the findings suggest that eating a varied diet early on in life—including early exposure to common food allergens—may actually be protective. One study comparing Israeli children with children living in the United Kingdom hypothesized that the earlier exposure of Israeli children to peanuts might account for lower rates of peanut allergies seen among these children.[7]

4. Finally, there is research examining possible links between trends in antibiotic use and the increasing incidence of food allergies and asthma that have been observed in some parts of the world. The increased prescription of antibiotics (and some other commonly used medications like acetaminophen) appears to parallel the rise in allergies and asthma, although a causative relationship has not been established. Researchers have proposed that early antibiotic use may change the intestinal flora. This could have an impact on the immune system's tolerance of potentially allergenic components found in certain foods. Other studies suggest that the increased use of acetaminophen may also be correlated with an increased risk of asthma and allergies.[8]

CAN FOOD ALLERGIES BE PREVENTED?

Although our understanding of allergic disease has increased, knowledge about the underlying triggers of food allergies remains an area of active investigation. There are likely several variables, both genetic and environmental, that influence the development of infant food allergies. There may even be environmental factors that influence the genes involved in the development of food allergies, so-called epigenetic factors.[9] In genetically predisposed children (those who have a first-degree family member with a food allergy), optimizing some of the known environmental variables may lower the risk of that child developing a food allergy.

Several studies have shown that exclusive breastfeeding for the first 4–6 months of age may have a protective effect in high-risk children—those with a parent or sibling who suffers from a food allergy. For high-risk children who are not breastfed, the use of a hydrolyzed formula, instead of a formula containing intact cow's milk protein, may also confer some protection.[10] Contrary to earlier scientific findings, delaying the introduction to solids beyond the recommended 4–6 months does not appear to prevent food allergies.[10,11] Breastfeeding mothers who have a family or personal history of food allergies should receive individualized advice from trained medical professionals on how to minimize the risk for their children. However, yet again, recent evidence suggests that the elimination of certain foods during pregnancy or breastfeeding may not play as large a role in protecting a child from food allergies as was once believed.[10]

FOOD INTOLERANCES

Some babies and young children can develop a condition in which they have difficulty digesting a given food—cow's milk is a common example. As a result of this, babies and children can experience symptoms like abdominal pain, bloating, and diarrhea. When adverse reactions to food are not mediated by the immune system, but rather by the digestive system, a child is said to suffer

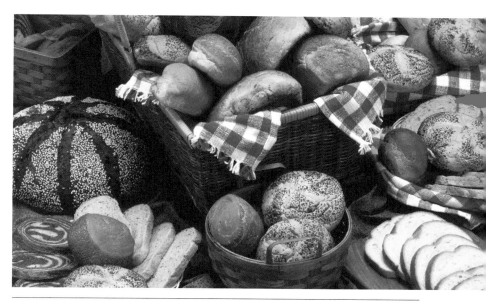

Figure 8.2 Celiac Disease is both an autoimmune disease and a food allergy to gluten found in wheat, rye, barley, and traditionally grown oats.

from a food intolerance rather than a food allergy. At present, our understanding of why some children are unable to tolerate certain foods, or how they grow out of this intolerance, is limited. Avoidance of poorly tolerated foods is the most common approach to managing childhood food intolerances.

CELIAC DISEASE

Celiac disease is considered to be both an autoimmune disease and a food allergy in which the allergen is the gluten found in wheat, rye, barley, and traditionally grown oats. In celiac disease, the immune system identifies gluten as a toxin, which, in an effort to defend the body, causes widespread inflammation and shedding of the villi lining the intestines. These villi are responsible for increasing the surface area for nutrient absorption; without them, an affected individual cannot absorb the nutrients in their food. The result is severe abdominal discomfort and diarrhea. In some affected individuals, a character-istic skin rash may also develop. As the child becomes deprived of nutrients, weakness and weight loss result, often to the point where the arms, legs, and buttocks become emaciated. At the same time, gastrointestinal bloating occurs secondary to widespread inflammation and malabsorption of nutrients. This can cause the abdomen to become bloated and distended. Malabsorption of iron and other nutrients leads to anemia, pallor, and weakness.

Diagnosing a child with celiac disease involves testing the blood for antibod-ies to some of the proteins found in gluten-containing grains. If these preliminary blood tests come back positive, an intestinal biopsy is performed to confirm the diagnosis. Many people experience significant symptoms of gluten intolerance, despite having normal blood test results when they are screened for celiac dis-ease. These individuals may sometimes also say that they feel better on a gluten-free diet and the term "gluten intolerance" is used to describe their condition. Increasingly, the gluten-free diet is being used as an adjunct treatment in the management of a variety of conditions in children, including behavioral condi-tions and autism. While many parents report improvements in their children on a gluten-free diet, scientific research in this area is still inconclusive.

Luckily, increasing awareness about celiac disease and gluten intolerance has made it easier to find gluten-free foods in many parts of the world. A healthy gluten-free diet includes a variety of naturally gluten-free foods, in-cluding fresh fruits and vegetables, dairy products, grains like rice, quinoa, millet, and buckwheat, as well as lean meats and fish. Gluten-free oats (that are grown and processed in environments free from contamination with wheat) can also be a staple part of a healthy gluten-free diet.

MANAGING FOOD ALLERGIES, INTOLERANCES, AND CELIAC DISEASE

At present, there is no known cure for food allergies, intolerances, or celiac disease. The primary treatment involves strict avoidance of the offending food in the diet and, for children who may experience anaphylactic reactions, ready access to injectable epinephrine and antihistamines for treating accidental exposures. The education of children, their families, and caregivers, including teachers, is also a key component of the successful management of food allergies and intolerances. Children and parents should know how to react in an emergency (especially for children with life-threatening reactions). Anyone purchasing food for the allergic child needs to know how to read food labels and identify ingredients that may pose a hazard. Similarly, anyone who prepares food for the child should be aware of the potential for cross-contamination and the importance of using separate utensils and food prep areas. For children with severe allergies, families need to be aware of the potential for exposure through routes other than ingestion of the allergen. For example, some children with severe peanut allergies can experience reactions from inhalation or skin contact with the allergen.

Hope for a Cure in Immunotherapy

A promising therapy, currently under exploration in the treatment of food allergies, is oral immunotherapy. To date, several studies have suggested that this form of therapy has the potential to reduce the severity of accidental food ingestion in most patients, and may provide a potential cure for food allergy in some patients.[12]

During oral immunotherapy protocols, children are exposed to gradually increasing amounts of their food allergen, under close medical supervision. This escalation of exposure in a controlled setting is continued until the child becomes partially or entirely desensitized to the food allergen. In most cases, maintenance of this desensitized state requires regular ingestion of a specific amount of allergen at home. In most cases, tolerance of the food allergen has proven more difficult to achieve than desensitization.[12] Tolerance refers to the state in which a previously allergic child can ingest their food allergen safely without having to consume a regular maintenance dose to maintain their non-reactive state. The safety and effectiveness of oral immunotherapy is still being examined and the factors that may lead to long-term tolerance are also still being assessed. Because allergic reactions can be life threatening, oral immunotherapy must be conducted under close medical supervision and should never be attempted at home. Even in a controlled setting, the safety of oral immunotherapy can still pose significant problems, with both mild and severe allergic reactions reported in most patients undergoing this therapy.[12]

Because food allergies can be life threatening, the diagnosis of a child with a food allergy can greatly affect the child's day-to-day life as well as the lifestyle of the entire family. Careful measures need to be taken to decrease the likelihood of accidental exposures while maximizing the child's confidence that their environment is a safe one, in which they can participate in the normal activities of childhood without hesitation or fear. Achieving this sense of security involves school and teacher awareness as well as ensuring that the home is safe and, ideally, free of allergens for the child. For children at risk of experiencing anaphylaxis, parents, teachers, and caregivers need to know how to administer an epinephrine injection and, once the child is old enough, they too need to understand how to act quickly in case of accidental exposure to the food allergen. Because of the increasing prevalence of nut allergies in recent years, many schools have declared themselves to be nut-free or nut-aware zones. At the very least, most schools will offer separate nut-free lunch tables for use by children who have severe allergies to these foods.

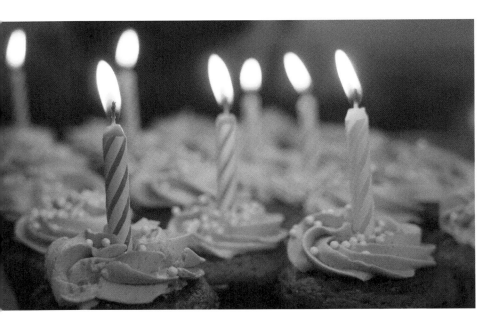

Figure 8.3 Helping a child to navigate social events involving food should be a priority in the management of a child with food allergies.

As part of the comprehensive management of the allergic child, the psychosocial implications of a food allergy or intolerance should receive ongoing consideration. Ideally, food restrictions should be implemented in a way that minimizes the child's interpretation of their allergy as a chronic illness. There are several ways in which this can be achieved:

1. Consider making the home an allergen-free (safe) zone for the child. When a child with a food allergy knows that everything in the home is safe to eat, this increases their sense of security at home. This also makes it easier for caregivers and guests, who may be less familiar with allergen avoidance, to keep the child safe.
2. When a child with a food allergy attends a birthday party or other social event where food is served, the potential for that child to feel excluded is high. Consider sending favorite, alternate foods for your child (for example, a homemade gluten-free pizza or nut-free cupcakes), ideally enough to be shared with non-allergic friends who might want to try some too. This allows the child to feel that they are sharing the pleasure of eating with friends, a key component of many successful social interactions.
3. Teach your child to cook! As soon as they are old enough to help mash bananas or shell peas, get your child involved in the kitchen. Teaching an allergic child how to prepare their favorite (safe) foods is incredibly empowering and can transform their food restriction into a celebration of the foods they love!

Parent Forum

Misha was a perfectly healthy boy until a few months after his third birthday. We had always noticed that his complexion seemed a bit paler than his two brothers, but his energy levels were excellent and he was growing and developing beautifully. Then one day, a week and a half before our family was scheduled to leave for a ski vacation, Misha developed diarrhea. Immediately, I started going over the foods he had eaten the days before the diarrhea began, but I could think of nothing unusual. So, I assumed my happy three-year-old must have caught a mild tummy bug and that this illness would pass. He had little appetite for food, but I made sure that he continued to drink and fed him small amounts of dry toast when he would accept it. Four days later, the diarrhea had worsened and we became worried. Misha's dad and I took him to our pediatrician, who examined him and assured us that this was probably a viral stomach bug—one that would likely resolve within a few days. We were advised to continue feeding Misha plain toast and bananas, with plenty of fluids, until the diarrhea stopped and we carefully followed this advice over the next few days. We assumed Misha would be well enough to enjoy the trip as planned and try skiing for the first time with his older brother. Instead, Misha and I spent most of our vacation in the hotel room, the diarrhea worsening instead of improving. My little boy was now beginning to look very pale and thin. Upon our return home, we went back to the pediatrician who wondered whether Misha might have caught a second gastrointestinal virus, thereby explaining the prolonged course of his illness. The pediatrician ordered basic blood tests and stool samples to be collected. Misha was found to be anemic, explaining his pallor, but the underlying cause of the anemia was still unclear. His stool samples also shed little light on what was causing his symptoms. Over the next few weeks, Misha's condition failed to improve and he became so weak that he scarcely had the energy to stand up on some days. We became increasingly worried, until my sister, a social scientist living in Canada, made a suggestion that seemed silly to me at the time: "Have you tried taking the wheat out of his diet?" she asked. I was hesitant at first—not believing that a food as ubiquitous as wheat could possibly cause such severe illness in a child. But, over the next two days, Misha was taken off the toast diet and fed only small amounts of rice. Miraculously his condition improved. Upon returning to the pediatrician yet again, we asked him if this could possibly be an acutely presenting case of celiac disease. I remembered learning about celiac disease in medical school, but had always assumed the disease would present more slowly, with chronic failure to thrive. The pediatrician agreed to test for the illness and Misha's blood tests came back strongly positive. He was suffering from an autoimmune reaction to the gluten found in wheat, barley, and rye, and to which oats are often exposed. An endoscopy with a biopsy of the small intestine confirmed the diagnosis. The walls of Misha's gut had been inflamed and damaged by his immune system's reaction to the gluten in his diet. This made it impossible for his body to absorb the nutrients in his food and explained his severe diarrhea, anemia, and weight loss over the past six weeks. The gastroenterologist reminded me that the only treatment for our son's disorder was lifelong adherence to a strict gluten-free diet. While the task of feeding our child safely seemed insurmountable at first, we slowly learned how to prepare foods that were not only safe and delicious for Misha, but also that the entire family enjoyed eating. Misha's father helped a group of young chefs start the first dedicated gluten-free restaurant in their area and the restaurant became a popular eating destination for many people who lived nearby—even those without sensitivities to gluten. Today, Misha is a happy, healthy boy who loves exploring new cuisines and knows how to read labels, ask questions, and determine whether or not a food will be safe for him to consume. He started learning to cook when he was four years old and could make gluten-free crepes (with supervision) by the time he was seven. When he goes to birthday parties, he always brings a tray of delicious, gluten-free treats to share with anyone who wishes to try them. More often than not, his friends say Misha's cupcakes are the best they've ever tasted!

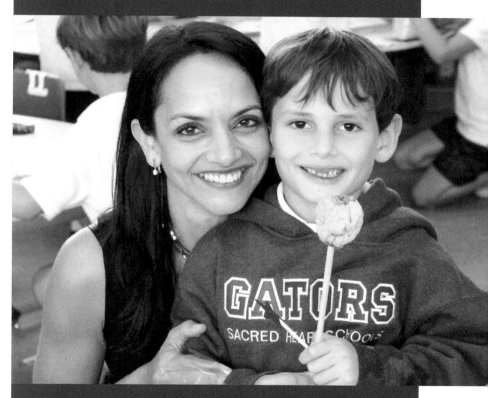

Figure 8.4 Teaching a child with food allergies to cook and read labels can empower them to stay healthy and enjoy their food, while minimizing anxiety.

CHAPTER 9

CHILDHOOD OBESITY

BY LAURA O'DONOHUE

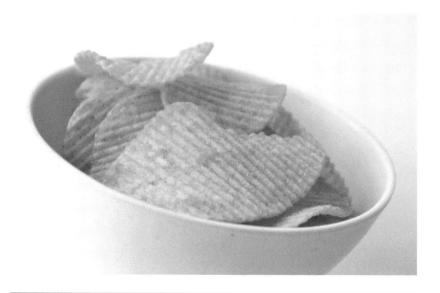

Figure 9.1 Potato chips are low in cost, but also low in nutrition and high in calories.

The obesity epidemic today represents one of the most difficult social and medical challenges confronting families and policy makers all over the world. In a single generation, some parts of the world have shifted from the struggle to get enough food on the table to a struggle to keep excess pounds off their waistlines.

Paradoxically, overweight and obesity are often intertwined with poverty and hunger.[1] Many are surprised to find that obesity can coexist with undernutrition or malnutrition. However, if food is low cost but high in calories, sugar, and refined carbohydrates, children and adults can easily exceed caloric needs for the day while failing to meet nutrient requirements.

WHERE ARE WE, AND HOW DID WE GET HERE?

Few countries have been spared the alarming rise in childhood obesity. In 2014, more than two thirds of the world's population was overweight or obese, and approximately 22% of those affected were children.[2] The increase in childhood obesity has been rapid. In 1970, 5% of US children were obese compared to 17% in 2008. That is over a 300% increase in less than 40 years. Obese children are much more likely to become obese adults[3] and this may be the first generation of children to live shorter lifespans than their parents due to obesity-related diseases.[4]

The obesity epidemic is often explained as a calorie imbalance: we take in too many calories and burn off too few. However, humans are complex biological systems, not simple math equations. Many factors, both genetic and environmental, can lead to childhood overweight and obesity and a variety of strategies can be implemented to prevent and treat overweight and obesity in children.

We are all exposed to foods and environmental inputs that have the potential to make us gain weight. These factors are often referred to as obesogens.[5] If these inputs are rare and moderate, such as a slice of birthday cake or the occasional poor night of sleep, they are nothing to worry about. When obesogenic habits and exposures become the norm, such as eating numerous pastries every week, or experiencing chronic poor sleep, significant weight gain can result.

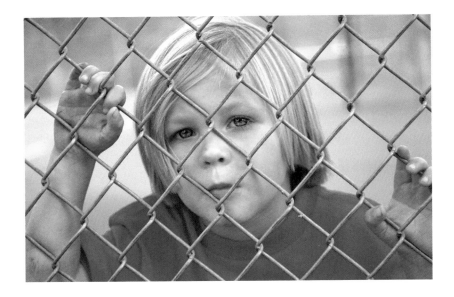

Figure 9.2 This may be the first generation of children to live shorter lifespans than their parents.

HEALTH RISKS AND COMORBIDITIES

DIAGNOSIS

The Body Mass Index (BMI) is often used as a rough assessment tool for a child's weight. The BMI is a mathematical equation that describes weight in relation to height.

$$\text{Body Mass Index} = \text{mass in kg}/(\text{height in m})^2$$

Table 2 shows a typical BMI chart. The United States Centers for Disease Control and Prevention defines overweight in children as above the 85th percentile and obesity as above the 95th percentile,[6] but percentile cut-offs for overweight and obesity are slightly different around the world.

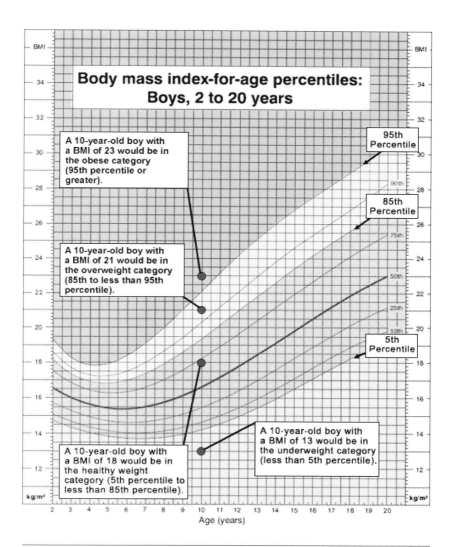

Figure 9.3 A body mass index chart is a helpful tool to determine if your child is a healthy weight for his or her age and height. BMI charts for girls, adults, and other age groups can be found at www.cdc.gov.

It is not only important to note how much a child weighs, but also where the weight is distributed.[7, 8] For an overweight or obese child who is active and growing, a reduction in waist circumference is a better indicator of progress than weight or BMI.[8] Waist circumference or hip-to-waist ratios are easily taken with a flexible tape measure and capture the amount of visceral, or abdominal, fat a child is carrying. Visceral fat is stored in the abdominal cavity around internal organs, which make it especially dangerous.[7]

There are healthy children who have evenly distributed weight and carry more muscle mass despite falling near the 85th percentile. Diagnosing these children as overweight may not be appropriate, as they may naturally grow into their weight as they get taller. Keeping a close eye on BMI *trajectory* and encouraging continued physical activity and healthy, long-term dietary habits can help assure the child stays healthy.

COMORBIDITIES

The chronic conditions that are caused or worsened by obesity are called comorbidities.

Obese and overweight children are at greater risk for comorbidities such as diabetes, heart disease, cancer, liver disease, hypertension, depression, sleep apnea, joint problems, and polycystic ovarian syndrome in girls. Table 3 lists many of the comorbidities of childhood overweight and obesity and their symptoms.[9] *Metabolic syndrome* is a common co-diagnosis of obesity. Metabolic syndrome is defined as the presence of three or more of the following five risk factors: a large waist circumference, elevated blood pressure, elevated blood sugar, low HDL, and elevated triglycerides.[10] Approximately 44% of obese children in the US suffer from metabolic syndrome, and many more are thought to have undiagnosed comorbidities.[11, 12] People who suffer from metabolic syndrome are also at increased risk of a host of diseases, including the common comorbidities of obesity listed above.

DIABETES

Diabetes is one of the most common comorbidities of overweight and obesity. To understand diabetes, we must understand the hormone insulin. Insulin is produced by the pancreas and its job is to help regulate blood sugar (or blood glucose). After a meal, blood sugar increases and insulin is secreted to help keep blood sugar levels in a narrow range for normal functioning.

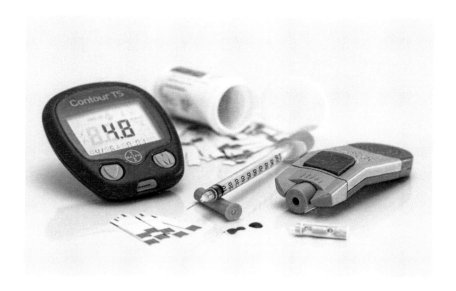

Figure 9.4 Diabetes is one of the most common comorbidities of overweight and obesity.

Blood sugar that is not used immediately for fuel is shuttled by insulin to our cells for storage, allowing us to maintain a narrow homeostatic window.

Diabetes is a disease characterized by elevated blood glucose. There are two types of diabetes: type 1 and type 2 diabetes. Type 1 is an autoimmune condition unrelated to weight, where the pancreas cannot produce insulin due to destruction of the insulin-producing cells. Once commonly called juvenile diabetes, type 1 diabetes can present in very young children.

Unlike type 1, type 2 diabetes is strongly associated with excess body fat and obesity. It occurs in older children and adolescents. In 1990, type 2 diabetes was rare in the pediatric population. Now more than 50% of adolescents with diabetes have type 2. This recent rise in childhood diabetes occurred in parallel with the increasing prevalence of obesity. Complex factors associated with obesity and the diets that contribute to it can render cells resistant to insulin, requiring the pancreas to produce more insulin to keep the blood glucose normal. Eventually, the pancreas cannot produce enough insulin to make up for the cells' resistance and blood glucose rises to an unhealthy level. When children exhibit excessive thirst, day- and nighttime urination, and mild weight loss without effort, an elevated hemoglobin A1c (HbA1c) or blood glucose test will indicate diabetes. Approximately 40% of children with diabetes will not have symptoms and must be diagnosed with laboratory testing.

DESIGNING A WEIGHT-LOSS PLAN

Action plans for achieving a healthy weight will vary depending on whether a child is still growing, the severity of a their current weight, and health risks. *Weight maintenance* is recommended for growing children who are moderately overweight, as they will ideally grow into their weight by adding inches more quickly than pounds.[13] If weight loss is necessary, it should not exceed 1 lb per month for children ages 2–5, and 1–2 lbs per week for children 5 and above.[9] Working directly with a health care provider can be very helpful to determine healthy and realistic weight-loss goals. Periodically measuring the waist circumference will also give a valuable measure of progress.

TURNING THE TIDE

EARLY CHILDHOOD

Obesity prevention can start in the womb. A mother's diet during pregnancy can influence the taste preferences of her children after birth. Amniotic fluid carries flavors of the mother's diet, and babies swallow many ounces of amniotic fluid every day. Mothers who eat a healthful, vegetable-rich diet in pregnancy are much more likely to have children predisposed to enjoying the complex, slightly bitter taste of vegetables as toddlers.[14] Additionally, research shows a strong correlation between breastfeeding and reduced risk of childhood obesity.[15] The benefits of breastfeeding are extensive and explained in more detail in Chapter 2. A mother's diet also impacts the flavors of her breast

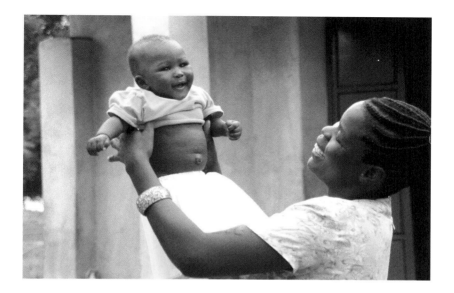

Figure 9.5 A mother's diet during pregnancy and breastfeeding can have an impact on her child's health.

milk. Tastes of a varied, healthful adult diet can prime children to eat and enjoy healthful, varied solid foods after weaning.[14]

NUTRITION AND DIET EXPECTATIONS

Weight loss can be a struggle for everyone, especially for children who may not understand the health risks of excess weight. If calorie reduction is needed for a child to achieve a healthy weight, it should be slow and moderate. The focus should be on reducing foods that provide little to no nutritional values. In other words, cut the chips, not the carrots.

One of the greatest sources of unnecessary calories is from sugary drinks, including soda, sports drinks, coffee drinks, and juices. There is a direct correlation between the earliest age at which a child consumes sugar-sweetened beverages, including juice, and future risk of obesity and disease.[16] Sugar-sweetened beverages (and artificially sweetened diet beverages) prime our palates and bodies for food. But these drinks don't deliver any nutrition, and the body is left craving more sugar and nutrients.[17]

After sugary beverages, one of the largest sources of calories in children's diets is snacks: candy, chips, cake, and cookies. When these snacks are replaced with more nutrient-dense whole foods, the body is able to register calorie *and* nutrient sufficiency, and hence real satiety.

The move away from junk food and sugary drinks can be challenging for children and adults alike. Some highly processed snack foods and sugary drinks, especially caffeinated sodas, have been shown to have addictive qualities[18] and are marketed heavily at those most vulnerable (as explained in Chapter 7). Slowly eliminating these foods from a child's diet may be easier than removing them all at once. There is no need to throw away the box of sugary cereal or donuts in your cupboard today. It's okay to take small steps in the right direction. However, once the junk food is gone, make sure to replace it with a healthier, real food alternative.

Severe calorie restriction or over-exercising should be avoided, *especially* for growing children. When we over-restrict calories, our bodies cannot tell the difference between a new diet and real food scarcity. This can trigger a hormonal response that causes an increase in hunger and a decrease in metabolic rate.[19, 20] It can be incredibly difficult to override this strong biological response when trying to adhere to a calorie-restricted diet. To make matters worse, severe calorie restriction causes both fat and muscle to break down.[21] With less muscle and a slower metabolism, it is much easier to regain weight in the form of fat as we resume eating a normal number of calories for weight maintenance.

Multiple unsustainable weight loss attempts can lead to yo-yo dieting, where the same amount of weight is lost and regained multiple times. Yo-yo dieting has lasting negative effects on metabolism, and should be discouraged in favor of whole foods, physical activity, and *moderate* calorie restriction over time, if needed.[22]

It is important that a weight loss plan thoughtfully address the environmental and psychological causes of excess weight, in addition to the role of calories. Childhood obesity is a complex issue and it is important to empower and support a child to make healthy decisions going forward rather than blame a child for their weight or past unhealthy habits.

BUILDING AN ENVIRONMENT OF HEALTH

EATING CUES

Children and adults are surrounded by environmental cues that encourage us to eat too much and move too little. It can be easy to finish an entire package of food, no matter the number of portions listed. It is tempting to sit all day when we are surrounded by computer screens. While changing these cues in a child's school may be out of your control, recognizing these cues in the home environment can empower families to make the healthy choice the easy choice.

Some of our eating choices are subconscious and are impacted by factors like plate size and how much we are served.[23] Our ability to know whether we've had enough is a combination of how full we feel and how we perceived our original portion size.[24] A normal-sized meal on a large plate might feel sparse. Take a look at the plates, bowls, and cups in your kitchen. Using smaller plates and filling them with appealing, healthful food can help promote healthier portions and eating habits.

SCREEN TIME

Screen time, not just sedentary time, is directly correlated to obesity in children and adults.[25] Besides the inactivity associated with screen time, children are much more likely to be exposed to advertising for unhealthy foods via screens. Screen time can also lead to mindless eating, or eating that is independent of hunger or even enjoyment of food. Many health and government organizations recommend less than two hours of screen time per day for older children and *no* screen time for children under 2 years of age.[26]

When a room contains television, TV will likely be the default activity in that room, so reducing screen time can be as simple as removing televisions and screens from all but one room. Given the demands of school, sleep, homework, and family activities, two hours of television, video or phone games can quickly consume any time that would otherwise be available for physical activity.

THE PARENTS' ROLE

Parents' and caretakers' commitment to offering healthy foods, regular meal times, and modeling healthy behavior themselves is one of the biggest factors in a child's successful weight loss.[27] Helping a child achieve a healthy weight requires working together as a family or in a parent–child partnership. Very young children do not go to the grocery store, purchase their own food, decide what's for dinner, and they certainly don't stop at fast food drive-thrus! Very young children also have trouble self-regulating their intake of highly palatable sweets and snack foods, so these foods are best avoided on most days of the week.

Efforts to offer healthier food are often challenged by children pleading at the grocery store for junk food, or on the way home to stop for fast food. Other parents and family members who do not understand or support your child's health goals may also pose challenges. If early challenges arise, that is OK! Research has shown over and over again that children (and adults!) learn to love new, healthful foods on repeated exposure.[28]

The easiest way to steer children toward healthy choices is to consistently present healthy choices. A useful strategy for the grocery store is to shop in the periphery, where the fresh produce and whole foods are usually displayed. By avoiding processed food aisles, children can be involved in choosing what to purchase (at least, to some extent), but their selections will likely be healthier foods. Instead of refusing to grant a child's request for an unhealthy treat, parents can try offering the child a choice of "healthier snack A or healthier snack B?" While being refused their favorite junk food might cause an adverse reaction the first time, a few experiences of leaving the store with healthier alternatives will quickly influence their willingness to enjoy healthier snacks and treats.[29]

Having a list of healthy snacks you approve of that your child can choose from *before* going to the store can help increase excitement about those items and prevent you from being distracted by others. Children are more likely to try something if they've had a role in choosing or making it. Try to engage children in other aspects of the cooking and meal-planning process, such as choosing which vegetable will be served, tossing the salad, or adding ingredients to a dish.[25]

Parental influence is more limited when children are older and have the what-and-when choices about their food. If weight is identified as a concern for adolescents and teenagers, it is important that they be committed to healthy

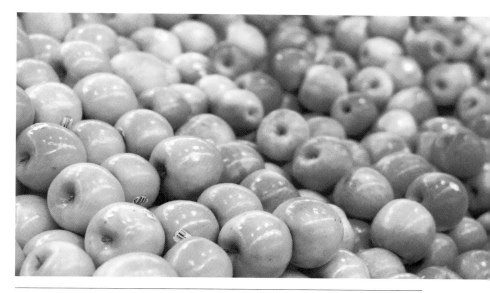

Figure 9.6 Making a grocery list with healthy foods on it before going to the store can help you and your family stick to a healthy eating plan.

changes along with the parents. It is helpful for the child and parent(s) to have clear commitments and responsibilities to each other in reaching new health goals. The parents' responsibility might be to stock only healthy items in the house that do not derail the child from their health goals. A child's commitment would be to stick to their health goals outside the home and be willing to try new healthy foods at home. Discussing health commitments with a health care provider in the room can give a sense of accountability to all parties and minimize the child taking changes personally or one parent taking changes less seriously.

REGULATION OF EMOTIONAL EATING

Regulating emotional eating, a desire to eat that does not stem from hunger, can be the most challenging but significant part of maintaining a healthy weight. Children inevitably model the behaviors of those around them, including eating behaviors of parents, siblings, and friends. Parents may have less control when older children are eating out with friends, for example, but the home remains the most important place to model healthy eating behaviors.

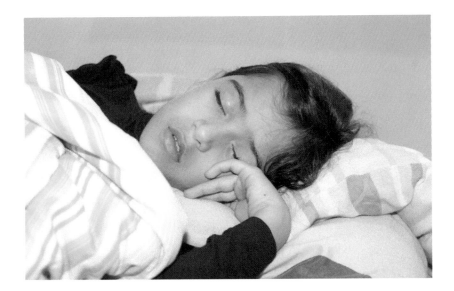

Figure 9.7 Adequate sleep is an important part of reducing stress and maintaining a healthy weight in young children.

Comfort foods are identified and internalized at an early age. For example, if candy is consistently given to a child as a reward or consolation, removing it from the diet may seem to the child like an undeserved punishment. When intimate family times and celebrations are linked instead with healthier foods (and even occasional treats), these patterns of food consumption are internalized and likely to be mimicked into adulthood.

Feeding your child healthy, nourishing food is a powerful and universal sign of love, and sweet treats have a special place at birthdays and holidays. On a daily basis though, there are many other ways to give comfort and positive reinforcement. Consider replacing food treats with other rewards, like choosing a family movie, reading a new book, or engaging in another favorite activity.

SLEEP AND STRESS

Research has shown that adequate sleep and stress management are critical to maintaining a healthy weight. Inadequate sleep can deregulate our hunger and satiety hormones, causing increasing sugar cravings and decreasing insulin sensitivity.[30, 31] In one study, infants who slept less than 10.5 hour per night were 45% more likely to be overweight at age 3.[32] In another study, researchers found that for every hour less of sleep a child got at ages 5, 7, 9, and 11, they were 50% more likely to be obese at age 32.[33] Children ages 1–2 should get 11–14 hours, children 3–5 should get 11–13 hours, and children ages 6–13 should get 9–11 hours of sleep.[34]

Perhaps the hardest aspect of encouraging sleep and stress management for children is modeling these healthy behaviors ourselves, so start with small but purposeful changes. Building up to slightly earlier bedtimes will take time, but the pay-off will be long lasting.

PLAY AND EXERCISE

When adults want to lose weight, they often visit the gym or engage in other forms of structured exercise. But children trying to lose weight can increase their activity levels through *play*. Activities like the monkey bars, basketball, hopscotch, soccer, biking, and running around the yard count as exercise too!

Do not let a lack of structure or rules discourage your children from engaging and delighting in movement. In fact, *unstructured* play with others may be the most beneficial for young children. While play and exercise may burn the same calories, the mental, social, and physiological benefits of play have been shown to outweigh solitary time on a treadmill.[35] The definition of play used here is *to engage in an activity for enjoyment and recreation rather than a serious or practical purpose.* Team sports are a wonderful way for children to play on a regular basis, but overweight children may be too self-conscious to enroll. In such cases, parents and caregivers should help the child to explore physical activities that bring them joy. It is important to provide *opportunities*, not just suggestions, for children to move. An easy place to start is a regular family walk, or other active family outings, like family bike rides along a bike-friendly route. This can be a time commitment for parents, especially if the child does not want to join an organized activity, but it is an invaluable investment.

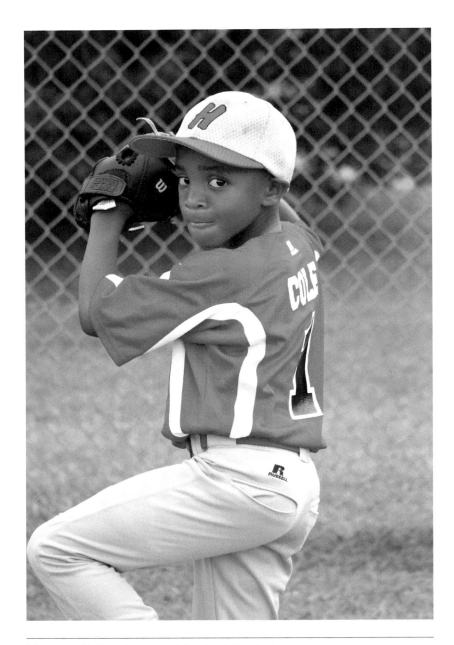

Figure 9.8 Physical activity should be fun!

CONCLUSION

We are just beginning to tease apart the causes of the rapid increase in child-hood obesity over the last 40 years. The childhood obesity epidemic is likely caused by a combination of factors, both genetic and environmental, but it is essential to remember that creating a healthy home environment for a child can trump environmental factors that work against their health. We are just starting to understand the incredible impact that our lifestyles and nutrition choices, possibly even more so than our genetics, have on our health.

Obesity and the chronic conditions that come along with it are especially hard on a child's growing body. Children with multiple chronic diseases will certainly not have the energy or ability to maximize their potential for leading full and happy lives. Childhood is the very best time to stop obesity in its tracks and turn the tide toward life-long healthy habits. Helping your child maintain a healthy weight does not demand perfection, but it does require progress, and that can start today.

CHAPTER 10

INTRODUCTION TO SUSTAINABLE FOOD

BY HANNAH KOHRMAN

WHY IS LOCAL FOOD BETTER?

"Local" food can have many different meanings: it could be food from your backyard, food from within 100 miles, or food from within the same state. A rule of thumb is that the closer you are to where the food was grown, the better. Fortunately, the movement toward local food is exploding. In the US the number of farmers' markets has quadrupled in the last two decades, and there are now more than 8,000 markets around the country.[1] In addition to farmers' markets and farm stands, many grocery stores carry local food in the produce section. So, why do we care about local?

BENEFITS OF LOCAL FOOD

- **Support your community:** One of the main benefits of local food is that it helps support your local economy, especially when you buy directly from farmers at a farmers' market, a farm stand, or a community supported agriculture (CSA) program. A recent study by the USDA showed that out of every dollar spent on food in the US, only about 12 cents goes to the farmer.[2] Most of the money goes to processing, energy costs, retail stores, and food packaging. The farmer gets a larger portion of your dollar spent at the farmers' market than one spent at the grocery store. The money you spend on local food stays in your community, instead of going to large corporations in other cities, states, or countries.

- **Freshness:** In general, local foods are fresher, since farmers usually harvest food the day before the market (or even the morning of!). Food grown nearby travels a shorter distance and takes less time to get to the market or store. This proximity of farm to market makes it more likely that the food is still at peak freshness and nutrient content. Additionally, fresher food often tastes better! Try a blind taste test with your children with a locally grown tomato or peach alongside the same produce grown as far away as you can find.

- **Carbon footprint:** Because local foods have traveled a shorter distance from the farm to your plate, they usually have a lower carbon footprint. Let's compare two apples: One was grown 50 miles away and driven in a truck to the farmers' market near you. The other was grown halfway around the world, stored in a shipping container, sent in a plane or boat to your city, and then driven to your market. The carbon footprint of the apple is a number that includes all of the greenhouse gas emissions caused by producing and transporting the fruit. While the true calculation is complicated, we can reason that the international apple has a larger carbon footprint and bigger environmental impact than the local apple.

- **Affordability:** Buying local food doesn't have to mean spending more. When you buy local food in the height of its season, it is oftentimes the same price as or cheaper than at the grocery store because the supply is large. When seasonal foods are cheap, it's a great idea to buy in bulk and preserve the food for later by freezing or canning. Some cities have worked to make local food even more affordable through programs that will double SNAP (formerly known as food stamps) money spent at farmers' markets.

- **Knowing where your food comes from:** Many people feel a deep sense of connection when they begin to learn where their food comes from. You can learn a new sense of time watching the season change through the changing foods, a new sense of place when you visit local farms, and a new community when you meet the farmers who grow your food.

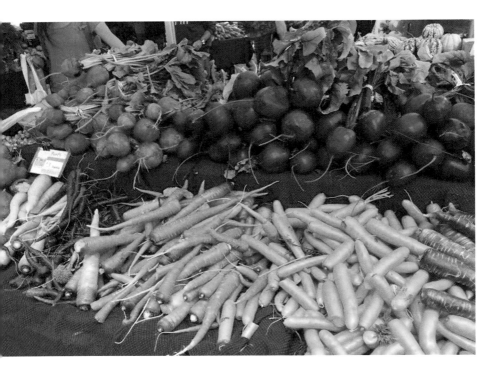

Figure 10.1 There are health, environmental and social benefits associated with choosing locally grown foods.

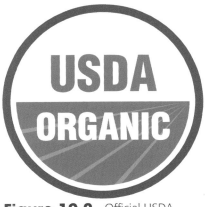

Figure 10.2 Official USDA Organic Seal

These reasons may inspire you to stop at a farm stand, visit a farm "U-pick" day, or do a local food taste test. Another way to have a steady supply of local food is to start your own garden. You can even enlist children to help with tasks like weeding and harvesting. Even if you only have a small balcony or windowsill, try planting a few herbs like basil or mint. Whenever you can choose local food, you make a choice for the environment, for your community, and for delicious seasonal produce.

WHAT DOES "ORGANIC" REALLY MEAN?

Organic is a term that describes the process of how food is grown on a farm. If food is certified organic, then it means the food was produced without synthetic pesticides, synthetic fertilizers, genetically modified organisms (GMOs), irradiation, or sewage sludge.

Why are these regulations important for the environment? In conventional agriculture (or "non-organic" agriculture), pesticides and fertilizers are used to help grow large amounts of food to feed billions of people. However, the way we use pesticides and fertilizers can have serious environmental and human health impacts. Sustainability issues associated with conventional agriculture include:

- **Greenhouse gases.** Fertilizers and pesticides are made from fossil fuels and are significant contributors to global warming. In the US, fertilizers are notoriously the largest contributor of nitrous oxide to the atmosphere. Consider that nitrous oxide is a greenhouse gas with 300 times the global warming potential of carbon dioxide![3]

- **Dead zones.** Oftentimes, farmers will administer considerably more fertilizer than plants can take up. This extra fertilizer runs off the farm into rivers and streams, and eventually ends up in lakes and oceans. Excess nutrients in the water can lead to dead zones where there is not enough oxygen to support marine life, resulting in massive fish kills. In 2013, the dead zone at the mouth of the Mississippi River in the Gulf of Mexico was larger than the state of Connecticut. There are more than 400 significant dead zones in bodies of water around the world, due largely to agricultural runoff.[4]

- **Pesticide resistance.** When farmers routinely apply pesticides to crops, it can lead to harmful pesticide resistance. The pesticide will kill the majority of pests in a population, but not the few that are able to handle large doses of the toxins. So, these stronger pests are the only ones that reproduce. When these pesticide-resistant pests reproduce for many generations, it can create superbugs that are fully resistant to the pesticides and can decimate entire crops.

- **Soil health.** A healthy soil is teeming with life: in one handful of organic soil there are more microorganisms than there are people on the planet! However, conventional agriculture relies on a suite of toxic chemicals to grow food, including pesticides, herbicides, and fumigants. These chemicals (which are banned in organic agriculture) can devastate populations of microorganisms in the soil, which are essential to the functioning of a healthy ecosystem.

Why is organic important for us? People choose to buy organic foods for a variety of reasons, when they have the resources and access. These reasons include reducing pesticide exposure in children, the public health threat of antibiotic resistance, and the harmful environmental impacts of conventional farming.

Community Supported Agriculture (CSA)

Subscribing to a CSA program is a great way to eat local and ultra-fresh produce, support local farmers, and try new kinds of foods. A CSA membership will get you a box of whatever fruits and vegetables are in season and at peak ripeness at the farm that week. A CSA subscription can save you time shopping and is often cheaper than purchasing the same foods from the grocery store. Some CSA boxes even include eggs, honey, meat, and flowers, and can include opportunities to visit the farm. Added benefits of CSA programs include ensuring farmers a steady income, taking advantage of seasonal bounties, and cultivating strong local markets.

- **Reduce pesticide exposure in children**. In 2010 the US President's Cancer Panel published a report recommending that, to the extent possible, people decrease their pesticide exposure by choosing food grown without pesticides or chemical fertilizers. Similarly the American Academy of Pediatrics calls for a reduction of toxic pesticide exposure in children. For many children, food is the most significant source of pesticide exposure. There have been many studies about pesticide exposure in farmworkers and children that show the potentially harmful health impacts of pesticides. Studies of farmworkers have linked long-term pesticide exposure to cancer, respiratory problems, depression, miscarriages, birth defects, and other issues.[5, 6] Other studies followed women who were exposed to higher levels of pesticides during pregnancy, and found their children to have lower IQ scores and poorer cognitive development than their peers.[7-9] The USDA regulates pesticide levels and confirms that levels of pesticides in conventional produce are very low and still safe. Even so, many parents choose organic to minimize any potential pesticide risk for their children.

- **Nutrient content**. There are conflicting studies about whether or not organic produce has more nutrients. Some studies show higher levels of nutrients and antioxidants in organic produce, and some studies show similar levels in organic and conventional produce. When nutrient levels are higher in organic foods, the explanation is likely because organic farming doesn't use pesticides. When there are no pesticides around, the plants are under more biological stress of predators and disease, so they have to produce more defense mechanisms to survive. The defense is made up of compounds called antioxidants, and these compounds are incredibly healthy for us too.

- **Reduce exposure to growth hormones**. Many conventional farmers use growth hormones to increase milk production in dairy cows or to help cows fatten up and go to market more quickly. One common growth hormone used to increase milk production is recombinant bovine growth hormone (rGBH or rBST). The FDA claims that levels of rGBH found in milk are within safe limits for humans, though rGBH is banned in Canada, Japan, Australia, and the European Union. Organic meat and milk will never contain growth hormones, and neither will food specifically labeled "No rGBH."

- **Foodborne illness and antibiotic resistance.** It is a fact of life that raw meat, whether it's organic or conventional, will contain bacteria. Proper meat handling and cooking are necessary to kill the bacteria and make meat safe to eat. But studies show that conventional chicken is significantly more likely to harbor strains of antibiotic resistant bacteria than organic chicken is, likely because of the overuse of antibiotics in conventional methods.[10] If someone were to get sick from bacteria on conventional meat, the foodborne illness could be much more difficult to treat. When possible, purchasing organic chicken will reduce your family's risk of exposure to antibiotic resistant bacteria, and will help support farmers raising chickens more responsibly.

It's important to remember that the term organic doesn't always mean that a food is healthful, especially if the food is highly processed. Just because a cookie is organic, it doesn't mean it's any better for us than the conventional version. But when it comes to the reasons above, we recommend that people choose organic foods when they have the resources and the food is available to them.

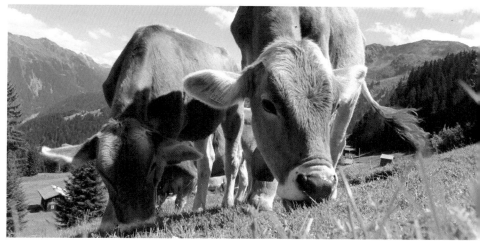

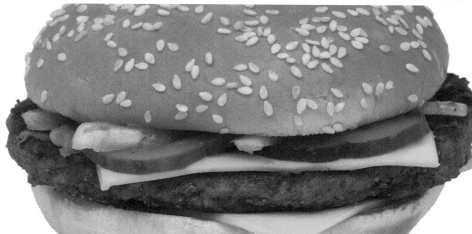

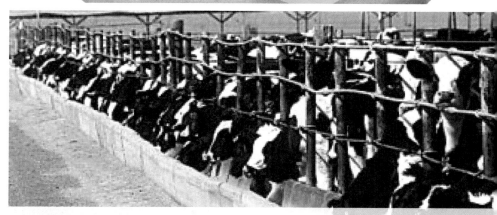

Figure 10.3. Where did the meat in this hamburger come from? What is the difference between cows raised in pasture or in Confined Animal Feeding Operations (CAFOs)?

MEAT AND SUSTAINABLE FARMING

The Global Footprint Network estimates that if the entire world's population lived like an American, we would need the resources of 4.5 Earths to support the global population.[11] It's fairly intuitive that driving large cars across suburbs and building large shopping malls are major contributors to America's high level of resource use. But it can be easy to forget that our diet actually has one of the biggest impacts on the environment. If we look closely at what we're eating, it is indisputable that the food with the biggest environmental impact is meat. Fortunately, it turns out that eating only moderate amounts of meat (or an entirely plant-based diet) is healthier for the planet and healthier for us too.

TRADITIONAL COWS

Over millions of years, cows evolved as incredible machines that transform sunlight into protein though an all-grass diet. Cows evolved to digest grass, a plant that is nutritionally worthless to humans since we can't digest it. Cows have a special stomach called a rumen, a four-chambered stomach filled with bacteria, which helps them break down and absorb the nutrients in grass.

The traditional food chain in cows is fairly simple: the Sun provides energy to help grass grow, cows eat the grass, and then cows produce manure. We call it a closed-loop system because there are no true waste products. The cow's manure is recycled as a natural fertilizer, and this manure is an essential nutrient source for the grass. Cows also help grass grow when they defecate in different locations, because they help spread the grass seeds in their manure and help plant the seeds with their hooves.[12]

MODERN MEAT PRODUCTION: "FAST FOOD"

In conventional livestock production, meat is raised very differently and involves many more inputs than just sunlight. Instead of eating grass, most cows today are fed corn. And instead of being raised on an open pasture, most cows are bred in factories called Concentrated Animal Feeding Operations (CAFO). A CAFO is essentially like a highly crowded city for cows, where tens or hundreds of thousands of cows are raised at a time.

Cows' shift in diet from grass to corn comes down to economics. Even though sunlight grows grass for free, it's cheaper to feed cows corn because the US government incentivizes farmers to grow lots of corn through subsidies. Additionally cows that eat corn require much less space—CAFOs are packed so densely they can produce thousands more cows per acre than a pasture. The last reason we feed cows corn instead of grass has to do with how cows metabolize corn. On a diet of corn, cows fatten up more quickly and can go to market more quickly. Historically, cattle raised on grass were slaughtered at around four or five years of age when they were large enough to go to market. Today, on a diet of corn, growth hormones, and antibiotics, an 80-pound calf can reach its 1,200 pound "market weight" in as little as one year.[13]

Meatless Monday

Meatless Monday is an international campaign encouraging partici-pants to go fully vegetarian for one day per week. This movement reminds us that our sustainability choices don't have to be all or nothing; just reducing the amount of meat we eat by one day per week can have a huge impact.

MEAT'S ENVIRONMENTAL COST

GREENHOUSE GAS EMISSIONS

The cheap prices of corn-fed beef don't take into account the enormous cost to the environment. A huge amount of oil and fossil fuels are needed to grow the corn to feed the hundreds of millions of cattle in the US. The fossil fuels are used to create the pesticides and fertilizers used to grow the corn and to power the tractors and machinery that harvest and transport the corn. Even more fossil fuels are needed to raise, process, and ship beef around the US and the globe. The fossil fuels used in every part of the industry are significant contributors to global warming; studies estimate that meat production is responsible for 14% of all greenhouse gas emissions.[14]

This graph describes the greenhouse gas emissions associated with the production of a variety of foods. To produce one kilogram of beef, 27 kilograms of greenhouse gases are added to the environment. For one kilogram of broc-coli or tofu, just about 2 kilograms of greenhouse gases are released into the environment.[15]

Some meat choices are better or worse for the environment due to differ-ent rates at which animals metabolize grain. For example, chickens are more energy efficient than cows are. Producing one kilogram (2.2 pounds) of beef releases almost four times the amount of greenhouse gases to the atmosphere as one kilogram of chicken. (And, because chicken has less saturated fat than beef, is better for your health too!)

Greenhouse Gas Emissions of Food

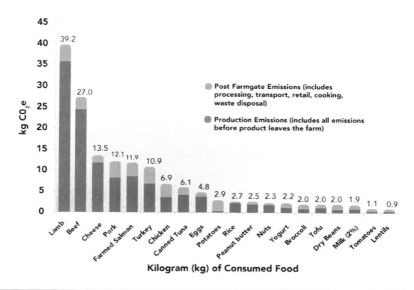

Figure 10.4 Plant-based foods have the lowest associated greenhouse gas emissions. When choosing between meats, chicken, turkey, and pork are more sustainable options than beef and lamb.
Source: www.ewg.org/meateatersguide

MANURE

Greenhouse gases are just one cost of meat. Another particularly offensive consequence is the amount of manure produced by millions of cattle. Where can it all go? Nowhere, really. So huge amounts of manure collect in enormous lagoons surrounding the CAFOs. Large quantities of manure can make it difficult to breathe for miles around, pollute nearby water sources, and reduce nearby property values.

ANTIBIOTICS

In the United States the vast majority of antibiotics are not given to humans to treat disease, but to livestock who may not even be sick. The Union for

Concerned Scientists estimates that 70–80% of antibiotics produced in the US go to livestock instead of humans.[16] Cows in CAFOs are more likely to contract and spread diseases due to poor diet, little exercise, and crowded living conditions. So, farmers feed them antibiotics before cows actually get sick to make sure they stay healthy. Also, giving cows antibiotics in their feed helps the cows put on weight more quickly (the mechanism is still unknown). If the cows get fatter faster, they can go to market faster.

But using antibiotics in large quantities is a controversial public health issue. Giving low doses of antibiotics to livestock selects for antibiotic-resistant pathogens. There is strong evidence that these pathogens can spread to humans through the food chain, and that it can be difficult to treat the illnesses. In 2006 the European Union banned the use of antibiotics for growth promotion.

WATER

Producing meat doesn't just take a lot of fossil fuels and corn; it also requires a lot of water. A food's water footprint is the number of liters of water it takes to produce the food, taking into account the water that the animal drinks and the water it takes to grow the food they eat over a lifetime.[17] Beef is one of the most water-intensive foods. To produce one kilogram of beef requires up to 15,000 liters of water[18] or enough water to fill about 88 standard bathtubs.[i] Eggs and chicken are protein sources that require significantly less water to produce than beef. As a comparison, most vegetables only require a small amount of water to produce, about 300 liters per kilogram.

One study compared the water footprint of meat-eaters and vegetarians. The researchers found that in industrialized nations, the vegetarians save about 1,300 liters of water per day, or reduce their total water footprint by 35%.[19] If we are interested in saving water, behaviors like taking shorter showers or washing our cars infrequently are a drop in the bucket compared to our dietary choices. By eating meat less often and choosing less-water-intensive meats like chicken, we can save thousands of gallons of water per year.

---

i   Assuming a standard bathtub holds 45 gallons or 170 liters of water.

WHAT IS SUSTAINABLE SEAFOOD?

Fish is a healthy and nutritious food that is high in protein, low in saturated fat, and rich in omega-3 fatty acids. Fish remains an important source of food in many traditional diets around the globe, like Japanese, Indian, Peruvian, and Caribbean cuisines. And there is wisdom in these diets: eating fish rich in omega-3 fatty acids is linked to a dramatically reduced risk of dying from heart disease, the leading cause of death in the world.[20] Fish consumption is important for pregnant women because omega-3 fatty acids are also beneficial for child brain and nervous system development. Additionally, eating fish has also been linked to lower risk of stroke, depression, and mental decline.[21]

But when it comes to fish, the sustainability rule of thumb that "what is healthy for us is healthy for the planet" gets complicated. Sometimes the fish that is healthy for us is damaging to the environment. Other times, toxins in fish could make it unhealthy for us.

ENVIRONMENTAL SUSTAINABILITY

A frightening statistic about fish: since the onset of industrialized fishing, 90% of global fish stocks have been fished to extinction or are in serious decline.[22] Simply put, overfishing describes catching so many fish that there are not enough fish left to breed and replace the population, so the population declines dramatically.

As global population increases, there are more people wanting fish as a source of food. Commercial fishing has grown tremendously to meet this demand; fleets use technology and more aggressive techniques to catch as many fish as possible, like using drift nets that are over a mile and a half long to catch fish. But by catching fish in significantly greater numbers, we're not giving fish enough time to breed and reproduce, so most fish populations are rapidly dwindling.

Another issue is that these long nets don't catch only the fish of interest; they can catch anything in the net's path, like turtles, dolphins, birds, sharks, and other marine animals. Fishing companies will keep the "prize" fish they can sell and dump millions of pounds of by-catch back into the ocean. These practices are highly wasteful, may eliminate key marine species, and can interfere with marine food chains. The Monterey Bay Aquarium estimates that in the shrimp industry, for every pound of shrimp that is caught, six pounds of by-catch are thrown away.

It can be difficult to regulate fishing practices, especially when considerable amounts of fishing take place in open international waters. But there is hope. In terms of policy, international groups are calling for global regulations to create catching limits, to establish underwater national parks known as marine protected areas, and to make it illegal to catch endangered fish. There is also hope on the consumer level. Resources like the Monterey Bay Aquarium Seafood Guide and the Marine Stewardship Council Certification help educate us on seafood issues and empower us to make sustainable choices.

HUMAN HEALTH

Scientists widely agree that the health and cardiovascular benefits of eating fish far outweigh the low toxicity risks.[21, 23] Since the health benefits of eating fish are great, doctors and scientists recommend that people eat one or two servings (about 12 ounces total) of fish per week and to minimize risk by avoiding fish high in toxins.

The human health concerns are that some types of fish may contain toxins that are harmful to our health when consumed in large quantities. The main contaminants that may be found in seafood are mercury, polychlorinated biphenyls (PCBs), dioxins, and pesticide residues.[24] These toxins are mostly the result of human pollution, and the toxins accumulate in fish that are high on the food chain, such as tuna and swordfish. Toxicity can be dangerous for people who eat a lot of these larger fish, particularly women of childbearing age, women who are pregnant or nursing, and children.

Guide to Mercury in Fish

High in Mercury	Low in Mercury
Tilefish (from Gulf of Mexico), Shark, Swordfish, King Mackerel	Salmon, Shrimp, Pollock, Tuna (light canned), Tilapia, Catfish, and Cod

AQUACULTURE: FARMED FISH

About half of all seafood sold in the world today is farmed raised rather than wild caught. Fish farming (also known as "aquaculture") is a rapidly growing industry that has the potential to increase the global supply of fish. However farm-raised fish may not be sustainable, and does not necessarily reduce pressure on wild fish in the ocean. Carnivorous fish species like tuna need huge amounts of wild fish in their feed. One study showed that up to 20 kg of wild-caught feed is needed to produce just 1 kg of farm-raised tuna.[25] It's more sustainable to farm herbivores like tilapia and catfish, since their feed is based on plant sources instead of wild fish. The overall sustainability of aquaculture depends on a variety of factors, including the species of fish being raised, how the system deals with waste, what the fish are fed, the use of antibiotics, and whether fish can escape into the environment.

Since the aquaculture industry is growing rapidly around the world, regulations vary significantly from country to country. Governments set different rules about the environment, social, and community considerations, and safety when it comes to farmed fish. Unfortunately there is not a one-size-fits-all answer to choosing sustainable fish, because it requires knowing the country's regulations and the specific industry. Independent certifications like the **Marine Stewardship Council (www.msc.org)** and **Monterey Bay Aquarium's Seafood Watch Guide (www.seafoodwatch.org)** can help us make environmentally sustainable choices depending on where we live.

When buying fish, the most important questions to ask are

1. **Where was it caught?** Location has a direct relationship to government regulations, sustainability practices, and social conditions for fishermen and processers.
2. **How low on the food chain is this fish?** Better to choose fish low on the food chain, because they will contain smaller concentrations of toxins.

3. **When was it caught?** The fresher, the better. (Another great option is fish that is flash-frozen at sea. Flash-frozen fish is preserved at peak freshness and nutritional quality and can be shipped by boat instead of plane, lowering its overall carbon footprint.)

SHOPPING SMARTS

The modern grocery store is a magnificent example of human progress: just 12,000 years ago we were only beginning to figure out agriculture, and today the average American grocery store contains more than 40,000 unique food products! With such a huge number of products, competition among food manufacturers to get us to buy their products is fierce.

Figuring out what food labels really mean can feel as complicated as deciphering ancient hieroglyphics. The mix of natural, free-range, cage-free, organic, local, and fair-trade labeling can be so overwhelming that we just

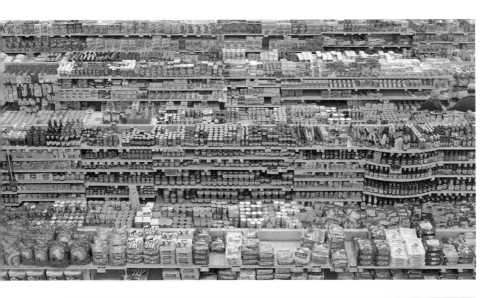

Figure 10.5 It can be difficult to make healthy choices in a modern grocery store.

grab the first thing on the shelf and make a run for it. Have no fear: in this section we're going to go over tips to help you be a smart consumer. We'll cover how to move through the grocery store, go over the difference between "natural" and "organic" (Hint: they're not the same!), and cover some of the most common food marketing terms. Knowing just a little bit about each of these terms can help you make informed choices and feel more comfortable when grocery shopping.

SHOPPING SMARTS

1. **Know your options.** Check your area for farmers' markets, farm stands, co-ops, and community supported agriculture (CSA) programs. Knowing all the options in your area can help you make informed choices based on budget, price, freshness, sustainability, and health.

2. **Take a shopping list.** A shopping list will make us less likely to succumb to the call of unhealthful food on sale that day, or candy in the checkout aisle. Also, sticking to a shopping list can help you stay within your food budget.

3. **Stick of the outer edge of the grocery store.** Have you ever wondered why the milk and eggs are in the back corner of the grocery store? Grocers have figured out that most shoppers enter the store for staples like milk, eggs, and bread. Stores are specifically designed so that getting to these basic items we need means we have to walk through hundreds of types of sodas, chips, and processed cereals. By sticking to the outer edge of the grocery store and steering clear of the middle aisles, we're more likely to pick up fruits and vegetables and avoid unhealthful foods.

4. **Know your labels.** As a rule of thumb, it's best to choose foods that make no health claims. (A head of broccoli has nothing to prove!) But a sugary cereal wants to convince you that just because it's low-fat, low-carb, gluten-free, vitamin-fortified, and mom-approved, it's healthy for your kids. (It's probably not.) In the next section we'll take a look at what these labels like cage-free and organic really mean.

5. **Reading ingredients lists.** If you baked a loaf of bread at home, you'd need some flour, salt, water, yeast, sugar, and a few other basic ingredients. But scan the back label of a loaf at the grocery store and you might find high fructose corn syrup, caramel coloring, stabilizers, and a whole slew of hard-to-pronounce chemicals. When it comes to ingredients lists, we like the common advice of "the fewer ingredients the better" and "only eat ingredients your great-grandmother would recognize as food." And again, the more items you can buy without a food label at all (like fruits, veggies, fresh meat, fish), the better.

NATURAL VS. ORGANIC

All Natural

"Natural" is one of the most misleading and over-used labels in the grocery store. The bottom line is *natural* means very little, and can often misguide consumers into thinking the food is healthier or more sustainable than it really is. The longer answer is wrapped up in more complicated government regulations set by the US Department of Agriculture (USDA) and the Food and Drug Administration (FDA).

The USDA says that for meat, chicken, and eggs, "natural" means that the food contains no artificial ingredients, added color, or synthetic substances, and is only "minimally processed." When meat is "natural," the animals can still receive antibiotics and growth hormones, and the label does not mean anything about farm practices, sustainability, or how the animal is treated.

The FDA does not define "natural" for fresh or packaged foods, so if the food does not contain meat or eggs, producers can essentially use the term however they'd like.[26]

Organic

Unlike the term "natural," the term "organic" carries a lot of weight because it is specifically defined and highly regulated. In the United States and in many other countries around the world, inspectors actually go from farm to farm to make sure that the organic standards are truly being met. Organic food is always produced without synthetic pesticides, synthetic fertilizers, genetically modified organisms (GMOs), irradiation, or sewage sludge.

Safety first! Best practices to avoid food poisoning

- Wash your hands and all cooking utensils with soap and hot water as soon as they come in contact with raw meat and poultry.

- Wash fruits and vegetables under running water before eating. (Do this even if you plan to peel the foods, because bacteria can still spread!)

- Keep hot foods hot and cold foods cold.

- Never thaw or marinate food on the counter; bacteria spread rapidly at room temperature. Instead, thaw foods in the refrigerator, microwave, or cold water.

- Don't wash meat, poultry, or eggs, because the splashing water might help bacteria spread to other parts of the kitchen. Instead, cook meat, poultry, and eggs to a high enough temperature to kill bacteria.

- Thoroughly cook meat, poultry, and eggs to kill bacteria, and use a thermometer to make sure the food reached safe minimum cooking temperatures (usually around 140° to 165°F or 60° to 74°C, depending on the type of food).

For more information, visit http://www.FoodSafety.gov

GROCERY STORE ENCYCLOPEDIA

BREAD: When shopping for bread at the grocery store, it's most important that the bread is **100% whole grain or 100% whole wheat**, meaning that it contains all of the nutritious parts of the grain kernel, including the bran and germ where most of the fiber, vitamins, and minerals are located. Don't fall for terms like "wheat flour" (not 100% whole wheat flour), "multi-grain," "natural," or "stone ground."

- Look for

    - **100% Whole Grain**: uses the whole part of the grain kernel, which maximizes the nutrients in the bread. Additionally whole grain breads are higher in fiber, which helps slow digestion and keeps you full longer.

    - **100% Whole Wheat Flour**: will be the first ingredient listed on bread that contains all parts of the grain. Beware that the terms "wheat flour" or "enriched bleached flour" mean the bread is mostly made of white flour, not whole wheat.

- Misleading Marketing

    - **Multi-grain:** beware of marketing! Multi-grain means that the bread contains more than one type of grain, but these grains do not have to be whole grains.

    - **Stone-ground, 100% natural, seven-grain, enriched bleached flour, wheat flour, (not whole wheat flour):** Beware of these marketing terms, which do not mean the bread is "100% whole grain or whole wheat."

    - **Caramel coloring**: check the ingredients list for caramel coloring, a food coloring that may contain carcinogens and should be avoided. Sometimes manufacturers add coloring to make enriched white flour appear to be whole wheat.

EGGS: If you were to choose one important label for eggs, "organic" is likely the most important. Organic eggs are free from antibiotics, and they are also cage-free and free-range. (Note that cage-free and free-range eggs that are *not* organic can still receive antibiotics.) Don't fall for the term *natural*, because all eggs are natural so the label doesn't mean anything. And if you care about animal welfare, look for Certified Humane, Animal Welfare Approved, or American Humane Certified.

- **Natural:** Does not mean anything! All eggs are natural.

- **Farm Fresh:** Does not mean anything.

- **Organic**: Hens were fed 100% organic feed and were not given growth hormones, antibiotics, or other drugs. Hens may not live in cages and must have access to the outdoors.

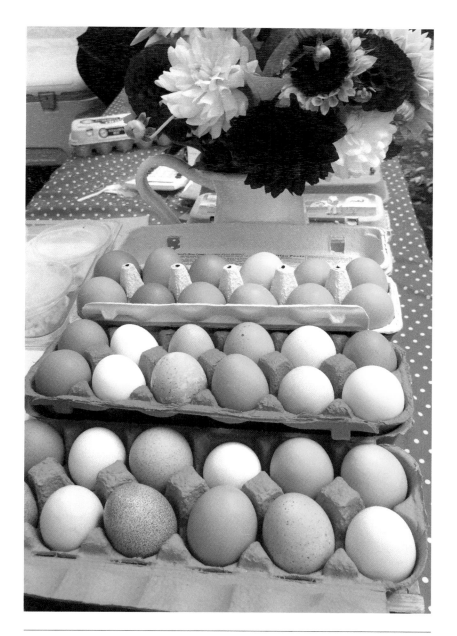

Figure 10.6 Try to choose organic eggs when possible. (And remember there is no nutritional difference between white, brown, and other colored eggs!)

- **Cage Free:** Means that hens are not confined to cages in the chicken house, but they may or may not have access to the outdoors. The term does not mean the hens were fed organic feed, and they may still receive antibiotics.

- **Free Range:** Means that hens are not caged and have continuous access to the outdoors. (While they have access, they do not have to be outside for a minimum amount of time.) The term does not mean the hens were fed organic feed, and they may still receive antibiotics.

- **Omega-3 Fatty Acids:** All eggs naturally contain a small amount of omega-3s, but this marketing claim usually means the hens were fed a diet enriched with omega-3 oils. Instead of paying the premium for omega-3 enriched eggs, we recommend getting your omega-3s from fatty fish like salmon, flax seeds, or fish oil.

- **Vegetarian Fed:** Chickens are not naturally vegetarian, since they eat worms and bugs. But vegetarian-fed eggs come from chickens who eat a special feed that does not contain animal by-products that can be found in conventional feed, like chicken litter, dried blood, feather meal, or ground-up poultry, meat, or fish.

- **Pasteurized:** Means the eggs are heated to kill any harmful pathogens found on the shell (but not to a high enough temperature to cook the eggs). Pasteurized eggs are useful for recipes that call for raw eggs, or for people vulnerable to illness.

- **Brown (or any color) eggs:** There is no nutritional difference between brown and white eggs, but many people think brown eggs are healthier than white eggs, like brown rice versus white rice. The color of the shell only has to with the variety of chicken laying the egg. Some hens lay blue, green, pinkish, and speckled eggs! Brown eggs usually cost more, either because the eggs are larger or because consumers think they are healthier.

POULTRY AND MEAT

- **Grass-fed beef**: means animals get most of their nutrients from grass throughout their lives. Unless also labeled Organic, or certified by the American Grass-Fed Association or the Animal Welfare Approved

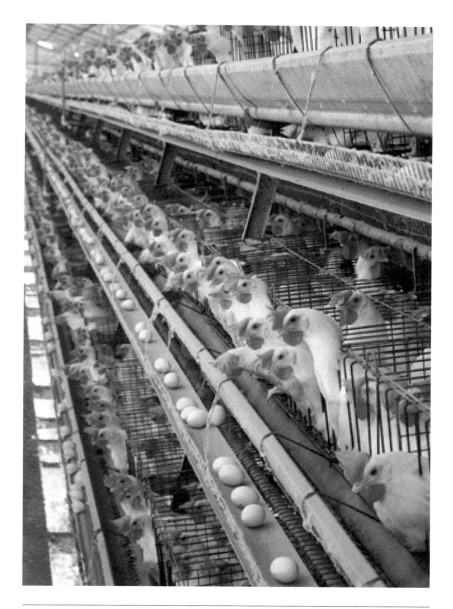

Figure 10.7 Many have welfare concerns about battery cages, which are commonly used in conventional agriculture. If you are interested in animal welfare, look for the humane certifications "Certified Humane", "Animal Welfare Approved", and "American Humane Certified."

Group (AWA), grass-fed animals may be given antibiotics, hormones, and insecticides. Grass-fed beef is more healthful than grain-fed beef: grass-fed cattle are lower in bad fats (like saturated fat) and higher in good fats (grass-fed beef has a healthier ratio of omega-3 to omega-6 fatty acids).[27]

- **Pasture raised:** the term implies that chickens and cows spent their lives foraging on pasture, but there is no official definition or regulation of this term by the USDA.

- **No antibiotics added:** as described, no antibiotics were used in production.

- **No hormones added:** may be used on beef labels if no hormones were used. Cannot appear on poultry or pork labels because hormones are never allowed in their production.

- **Natural:** essentially means nothing. Defined as "no artificial ingredients; minimally processed."

HUMANE CERTIFICATIONS

- **Certified Humane, Animal Welfare Approved, and American Humane Certified:** These are some of the most widely recognized humane certifications. Third-party auditors visit the farms to make sure the standards are being met. These certifications cover a variety of welfare issues like cages, antibiotics, beak trimming, forced molting, and animal by-products in feed. Depending on which country you live in, there may be other humane certifications present on labels.

Every time we spend a dollar on food, we are voting with that dollar. We send a message through the market about our values and preferences, and what we support. So when you are able, try to buy local, organic, and sustainable food more often. It will be good for you, your children, your community, and your environment.

CHAPTER 11

PRENATAL NUTRITION

For many women, the experience of creating new life brings with it a newfound respect for the capabilities of the human body. The changes that occur during pregnancy and birth can seem both astonishing and miraculous to an expectant mother. As natural as this process is, the building of a baby human inside the adult human body is a complex biological task. It relies both on carefully timed biological stimuli and the availability of specific building blocks. Many of those building blocks come from the mother's diet. Simply put, babies are built from food. Taking in the right quantity of food and maximizing the nutritional quality of that food is an important way in which a pregnant woman can support the development of a healthy child. Mothers who are educated and motivated to make healthy food choices, *before* their babies are born, really are laying the foundations for their own future health and the health of their children.

The choices parents make about what to eat have ongoing, lifelong implications for their children, but for a mother, eating well during pregnancy may be more important than at any other time. Sensible prenatal food choices do more than support the growth and development of the fetus. They may end up actually influencing the taste preferences and future food choices of the child.[1-3] These early preferences are powerful contributing factors to the lifelong health of a child. By exposing the developing fetus to a variety of healthy foods in utero, a mother can begin caring for her baby long before birth.

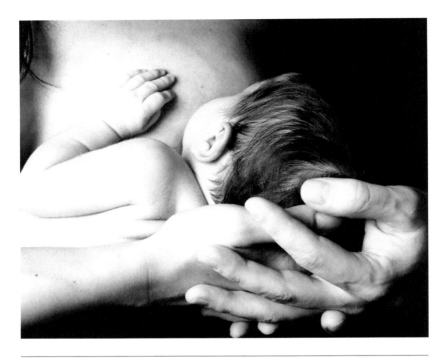

Figure 11.1 Future food preferences may be shaped through exposure to flavors in utero and during breastfeeding—long before a baby takes her first bite of solid food.

Scientific research suggests that babies may actually begin sampling food before they're born. Through the amniotic fluid, the fetus may sense and become accustomed to the flavors of foods eaten by the mother. This subtle flavor sampling continues throughout breastfeeding and sets the foundation for a child's future food preferences. When a pregnant woman's diet is sufficiently varied, her baby is more likely to be accepting and open to a variety of foods later in life. A breastfeeding mother's diet likely has a similar influence on the flavors her infant experiences during breastfeeding.[1-3] This means that future eating habits are potentially being shaped long before our babies take their first bite of solid food—yet another reason for pregnant women and new mothers to eat a balanced and varied diet. Early flavor experiences prepare a baby for her earliest encounters with solid food, allowing her to enjoy the richness of flavors the world has to offer.

WHAT TO EAT DURING PREGNANCY

In general, the best advice on what to eat during pregnancy is closely aligned with the general health messaging in this book. Healthy pregnant women should ideally eat a variety of fresh, wholesome foods, in moderate quantities, ideally in a stress-free, safe environment. A healthy pregnancy diet looks a lot like a healthy regular diet—with plenty of fresh fruits and vegetables, good sources of protein, whole grains, and a moderate amount of healthy fats, like

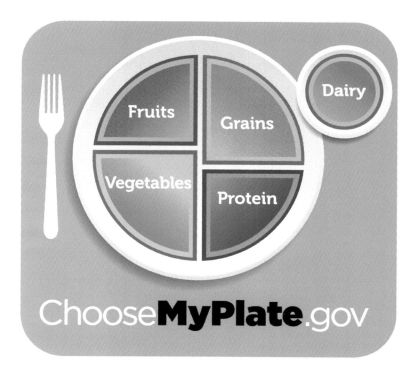

Figure 11.2 The USDA MyPlate icon was released by the US Government in 2011.

those found in avocados and olive oil. In general, and in line with current USDA recommendations,[4] a healthy meal for a pregnant woman is made up of approximately one half plant-based foods, one quarter lean protein, and one quarter unrefined, whole-grain carbohydrates. For some ideas and specific examples of appropriate foods, see the image and table below.

Healthy Prenatal Diet

Examples of foods that can be included in a healthy prenatal diet

Vegetables	Fruits	Grains	Proteins
Carrots	Oranges	Brown rice	Eggs
Broccoli	Apples	Whole wheat pasta	Kidney beans
Squashes	Pears	Quinoa	White beans
Lettuce	Peaches	Millet	Lentils
Cucumbers	Pineapples	Teff	Nuts
Peppers	Mangos	Sorghum	Split peas
Cauliflower	Grapes	Oats	Garbanzo beans
Eggplant	Lemons	Cornmeal	Tofu
Mushrooms	Limes	Whole wheat bread	Fish
Onions	Lychees	Buckwheat	Chicken
Garlic	Bananas	Farro	Lean red meats
Fresh herbs	Berries		Dairy products

WHAT NOT TO EAT (OR DRINK) DURING PREGNANCY

ALCOHOL

The link between heavy maternal alcohol consumption during pregnancy and various adverse birth outcomes has been well established.[5, 6] Alcohol consumption during pregnancy has been linked to an increased risk of babies being born preterm, having low birth weight, and being small for gestational age. Studies have also shown that heavy alcohol consumption during pregnancy may be associated with later behavioral issues in the child.[7] The effects of low to moderate alcohol consumption during pregnancy are less clearly understood and the scientific findings in this area are not definitive,[8-12] so it is generally considered to be safest for pregnant women to avoid alcohol entirely during pregnancy.

FOODS TO AVOID

Like many of the fetal body systems, the immune system is a work in progress during pregnancy. This system, designed to eventually help fight off infections, is underdeveloped while the fetus is inside the womb. As a result, the fetus is more vulnerable to pathogens than is an older baby or young child. To some extent, the fetus is protected by the mother's immune system, but there are certain foods that may carry an increased risk of foodborne infections. Some women choose to avoid these foods entirely during pregnancy, although the absolute risks associated with them may be small. It's important to remember that, for the most part, these are recommendations rather than directives. More than any single food, the thing that should probably be avoided most consistently during pregnancy is excessive stress—including the stress that can result from a fear of eating the wrong foods! Having said that, here are some of the foods that pregnant woman may want to minimize or avoid entirely.

- **Soft cheeses**. Soft cheeses made from unpasteurized milk can harbor bacteria that, in some cases, may be harmful to the fetus. A few examples are brie, camembert, and roquefort. It may be wise to choose hard cheeses like cheddar or swiss, or to check the label on soft cheese and avoid those made with unpasteurized milk.

- **Undercooked animal foods**. It may also be wise to avoid rare meat; raw or undercooked fish such as sushi, raw oysters, and clams; raw cookie dough or cake batter, eggnog, unpasteurized eggs, unpasteurized milk, and unpasteurized juices. It's sometimes recommended that, during pregnancy, eggs be cooked until both the egg yolk and the white are firm. Processed meats like cold cuts, hot dogs, sausages, and other deli-style meats can also contain harmful bacteria. If these meats are eaten during pregnancy, they should be thoroughly reheated before eating.

- **Sprouts.** Raw or undercooked sprouts such as alfalfa or clover can also contain microbes that could harm the fetus, so these should be avoided, if possible, or cooked at high heat to kill any pathogens.

PREGNANCY CRAVINGS

An impressive collection of legends and fairytales include, as part of their storyline, the strange and powerful cravings of the pregnant woman. Rapunzel's father broke into a witch's garden to steal the Rapunzel plant when his pregnant wife's cravings for it grew so strong she thought she might die without it. Pregnancy, it seems, can make even the most rational woman (and even sometimes that woman's partner) go out of their way to procure specific foods. While many of these stories are anecdotal, there have also been several scientific investigations of the phenomenon.[13-15] In general, the findings show that a pregnant woman's body may be giving her feedback about the nutrient needs of the fetus. For example, there is research supporting the finding that some women develop cravings for sour foods, even if they weren't fond of these foods before becoming pregnant, potentially resulting in increased vitamin C intake. At the same time, some women who regularly drank coffee before pregnancy have reported an aversion to coffee during pregnancy.[15] Both the fairytales and the research findings imply that there may be a great deal of benefit for the fetus if the woman listens to her body as she tries to make sensible, educated decisions about the food she eats during pregnancy.

KEY NUTRIENTS DURING PREGNANCY

There are several important vitamins and minerals that play key roles in the development of a healthy fetus. Let's discuss those here:

Folic acid is widely recognized as an important nutrient for a pregnant woman and her growing fetus. This vitamin plays an important role in both growth and maintenance of the mother's placenta and in fetal neural development.[16] Folic acid is found in dark, leafy greens, whole grains, nuts, legumes, and oranges. Many physicians recommend a folic acid supplement for women who are planning a pregnancy. However, women of childbearing age who lack access to folic acid supplements can get enough of this important nutrient by eating a well-balanced diet, including foods rich in folic acid.

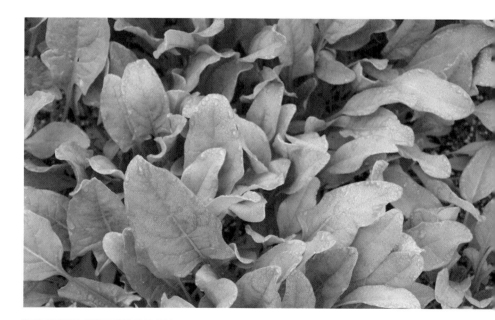

Figure 11.3 Spinach is an excellent source of folic acid, an important nutrient during pregnancy and fetal development.

Iron is another important nutrient for supporting the rapid growth that occurs during a healthy pregnancy. This mineral is a key component of the blood protein hemoglobin, which helps to carry oxygen around the body. During pregnancy, a woman without enough iron may develop a condition known as iron-deficiency anemia, which can increase the risk of delivering a small or preterm infant. Infants born with iron deficiencies are also at higher risk of experiencing developmental delays.[17] Meats (especially red meat, dark turkey meat, and organ meat, like liver and kidney) are excellent sources of iron. The iron found in these animal-based foods is called *heme* iron. A somewhat less-efficiently absorbed form of iron (*non-heme* iron) is found in many plant-based foods (including beans, almost all other legumes, and even spinach). The absorption of *non-heme* iron is enhanced when these plant-based foods are combined with foods rich in vitamin C or with any form of meat, poultry, or fish.[18]

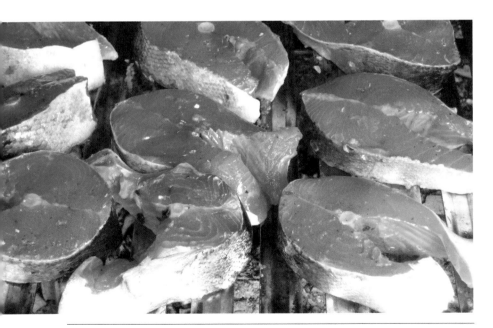

Figure 11.4 Salmon is a sensible choice for pregnant women who want to eat fish because it is a good source of omega-3 fatty acids and lower in mercury than some other fish.

For pregnant women, eating moderate amounts of fish on a weekly basis may have additional benefits because fish oil contains essential omega-3 fatty acids, which may be important in supporting healthy fetal brain development.[19] However, it's important to keep in mind that some fish, especially large predatory fish like tuna and swordfish, can also contain dangerously high levels of mercury. Consuming excessive amounts of these fish during pregnancy could have harmful effects on the fetus.[20] For pregnant women, good choices for a once- or twice-a-week fish dish are salmon, herring, and trout, among others. (You can find more on fish and seafood in Chapter 10.)

IODINE

In many parts of the world, iodine deficiency is still a major cause of concern during pregnancy.[21] In areas of severe iodine deficiency, the risks of serious health problems for both the iodine-deficient mother and her fetus have led to urgent calls for iodine supplementation.[22] In the United States and many other countries, iodine is added to table salt, which has nearly eliminated iodine deficiency. Iodine deficiency during pregnancy remains a serious problem in parts of the world where it is not readily available in the diet.[23]

VITAMIN D AND CALCIUM

During pregnancy, changes in maternal metabolism of vitamin D and calcium allow the woman's body to provide the calcium needed for fetal bone development. By the end of a healthy pregnancy, 25–30g of calcium are transferred from mother to fetus, most of this occurring during the third trimester.[24] Vitamin D plays an important role in the absorption of dietary calcium and it can be obtained through the diet (from fortified milk, fatty fish, and eggs, for example) or through exposure to sunlight.

Women who do not get enough sun exposure may be at risk for vitamin D deficiency. This is especially a concern during the winter months. In the United States, milk is typically fortified with vitamin D, which has improved vitamin D intake levels. In countries that don't fortify dairy products, and in cultures where women cover most of their skin, a vitamin D supplement may be recommended during pregnancy and nursing.

DO I NEED A PRENATAL VITAMIN?

Prenatal vitamin supplements can be used to *complement* a healthy diet but are not a *substitute* for good nutrition in pregnancy. A healthy diet is the best way to supply the mother and fetus with all the necessary vitamins and minerals to support a healthy pregnancy. A varied diet of fruits, vegetables, dairy products, whole grains, seafood, meats, legumes, nuts, and seeds should be the primary approach to achieving good prenatal nutrition. Since iron and folic acid are especially important, a supplement containing these (as well as a variety of other vitamins and minerals) is recommended during pregnancy for most women.

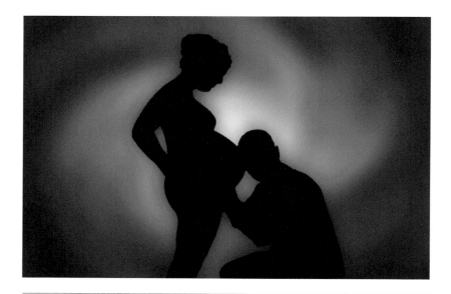

Figure 11.5 A balanced diet with plenty of variety should be the primary approach to healthy prenatal nutrition.

EATING VEGETARIAN OR VEGAN DURING PREGNANCY

Women who choose to eat a vegetarian or vegan diet during pregnancy need to give special consideration to a few nutrients that may need to be supplemented during pregnancy. Especially in the case of a vegan diet, pregnant women should pay special attention to making sure their daily meals contain adequate protein, calcium, vitamin D, iron, vitamin B12, and essential fatty acids. Combining plant-based foods (like beans with corn or lentils with rice) is an important and time-honored way of ensuring that the protein in a vegetarian meal is complete—that it provides all of the essential amino acids to support growth and maintenance. Other examples of complete protein combinations are brown rice and black beans, pinto beans and corn tortillas, dal and rice, or peanut butter and wheat bread. There are also some sources of plant protein, including quinoa, buckwheat, soy, and chia, that provide a complete source of protein without needing to be combined. However, eating a variety of foods has many other health benefits, including reducing exposure to any hidden toxins (like pesticide residues) that may be found in any single food.

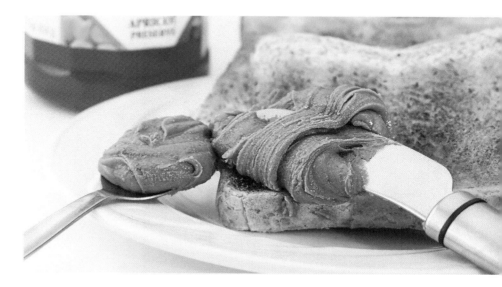

Figure 11.6 Peanut butter and whole wheat bread are an example of a complete protein combination.

ENERGY INTAKE AND WEIGHT GAIN

The caloric needs of a pregnant woman depend on several factors, including body mass index (BMI) before pregnancy, metabolic rate (the rate at which calories are used for energy), age, and activity level during pregnancy. Some women will enter pregnancy overweight or obese, while others may start off underweight. The Institute of Medicine (IOM) in the United States warns that, in general, "women today are heavier; a greater percentage of them are entering pregnancy overweight or obese, and many are gaining too much weight during pregnancy".[25] The 2009 IOM recommendations for weight gain during pregnancy, by pre-pregnancy BMI (see Table 10.1), are intended to guide physician recommendations for weight gain, diet, and exercise during pregnancy.

Prepregnancy BMI	BMI+ (kg/m²)	Total Weight Gain (lbs)	Rates of Weight Gain* 2nd and 3rd Trimester (lbs/week)
Underweight	<18.5	28–40	1 (1–1.3)
Normal weight	18.5-24.9	25–35	1 (0.8–1)
Overweight	25.0-29.9	15–25	0.6 (0.5–0.7)
Obese (includes all classes)	≥30.0	11–20	0.5 (0.4–0.6)

+ To calculate BMI go to www.nhlbisupport.com/bmi/
* Calculations assume a 0.5–2 kg (1.1–4.4 lbs) weight gain in the first trimester (based on Siega-Riz et al., 1994; Abrams et al., 1995; Carmichael et al., 1997)

Figure 11.7 New recommendations for total and rate of weight gain during pregnancy, by pre-pregnancy bmi.

It is also important to note that weight gain beyond the IOM recommendations has been associated with an increased risk of the child becoming overweight or obese.[26] While specific recommendations for prenatal nutrition vary somewhat around the world, pregnant women will probably need between 2,000 and 2,900 calories a day. In the United States, the American Dietetic Association recommends no additional calories per day in the first trimester, 340 additional calories per day in the second trimester, and 450 additional calories per day in the third trimester.[27] Many women are surprised how quickly the additional recommended 340–450 calories can be consumed. A standard peanut butter sandwich and an apple would suffice!

IN CONCLUSION

Just like teaching a child to read, the process of teaching a child to enjoy a variety of healthful foods requires patience and gentle perseverance. Today, parents are increasingly advised to read to their children even before they seem to understand the words that are being read to them. Similarly, we can expose our children to the right foods even before they are ready to eat them. By doing the best we can to make healthy choices from the foods that are available to us, we can expose our children to a wide variety of fresh, wholesome flavors, setting them up for a lifelong love affair with real, delicious food.

CHAPTER 12

A CALL TO ACTION: JUST COOK

Here in the United States, and increasingly around the world, our children are facing an epidemic of chronic disease that threatens to leave them with a shorter life expectancy than their parents. The disease is childhood obesity and the increasing amount of processed food in the typical Western diet is one of the biggest culprits. Parents and caregivers often find themselves battling to raise healthy children in what has been described as an obesogenic food environment—an environment that sets our children up for disease instead of good health. In parts of the world where processed food is ubiquitous, powerful food marketing forces subtly influence parents and children from street corners, billboards, magazines, and screens. School cafeterias that continue to offer highly processed food reinforce these choices as appropriate ones in the eyes of the next generation. The increasingly sedentary nature of childhood, in many parts of the world, confounds this global public health crisis.

Many children around the world are struggling with overweight and obesity because the responsibility of feeding them has been taken away from loving parents and caregivers. The increasing availability of packaged foods has made it easy for parents to avoid the kitchen altogether. Gradually, many parents have become convinced that they don't have the time, money, or skills to feed their families. In some communities, cooking is regarded as an activity reserved for celebrity chefs—not to be attempted at home by amateurs. Agricultural food subsidies, coupled with longer working hours and tighter budgets, have helped make the production of highly processed convenience food into a profitable business for many food producers. As children witness their parents' own struggles to choose healthful, balanced foods, a cycle of unhealthy eating and mixed emotions about food can all too easily be passed on to the next generation.

The foundations of a child's relationship with food are important to protect. In decades past, when societies around the world were more intimately connected with the production of their own food, eating was seen as a community-building, celebratory activity. With the rise of processed food consumption, and the parallel increase in obesity and other associated chronic diseases, eating has become a potentially threatening activity. Instead of naturally supporting

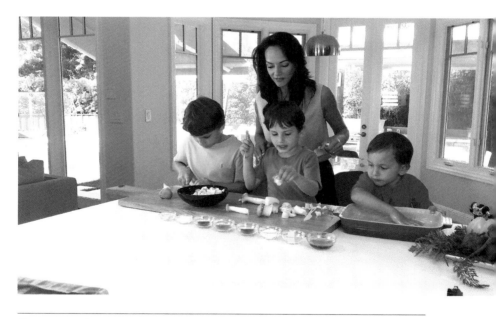

Figure 12.1 Cooking together can help to strengthen the foundations of our children's relationship with food, while protecting their health.

our good health, it often seems that too many unhealthy foods are out there to tempt us to deviate from our health goals. Yet, in an obesogenic food environment, placing the blame on the individual is both unfair and unproductive.

While the origins of our problem may be complex, the solution doesn't have to be. We need to start cooking again. When we cook at home, we regain control over the food our families eat. Fast food companies prioritize short-term profits over the health of the next generation. If we can reallocate a small amount of time and money toward simple home cooking, we take back the reins. Our kitchen pot is a powerful tool in the fight against childhood obesity because the person deciding what to put in it has a vested interest in the quality of the product. Above and beyond the improvements in nutritional content, there's a lot to be gained when a parent or trusted caregiver becomes the most familiar source of food.

WHY DO I COOK?

Families around the world treasure their children from the moment they are born. Like most parents, my children are as important to me as the air that I breathe, so I am writing these words for them. I believe that we can transform the landscape of food that currently forms the backdrop of childhood in too many parts of the world, and the increasing encroachment of processed food into other parts of the world. We can shape our eating environment into one that supports our children's health and allows us all to stop fearing food, because we've learned to love the right food. Meal by simple meal, we can reboot the culture of eating and redefine our children's comfort foods to be the ones that will truly comfort them throughout the full and healthy lives that they deserve.

My lack of formal training in the culinary arts is just one of the reasons that I do not claim to be a gourmet cook. But, like many of you, I am raising children in a food environment that puts their health at risk. Cooking can reduce that risk.

So, I cook because I have to. Because I know how dangerous it is NOT to cook, because I want to raise children who know that an artichoke is not a wrestling tactic—children who will one day be able to prepare a simple pasta dish with fresh tomato sauce when they are alone in their first bachelor pad. But those aren't the only reasons I do it. I also cook for that look in their eyes when they see me getting out the eggs and a big silver bowl. I cook so they will come running, yelling, "Can I help? Can I be the egg-cracker?" I cook so there's an excuse to reconnect at the end of a long day and to celebrate each week with our family and friends. I cook so we will stay together, stay healthy, and be aware of our gifts. I cook because I love.

ASPARAGUS TORTA

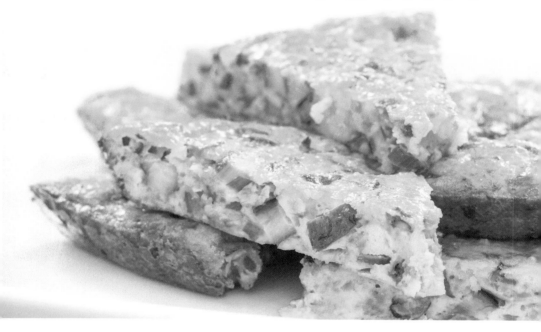

INGREDIENTS

½ bunch of fresh asparagus

½ onion, chopped

1 garlic clove

4 eggs

¼ cup panko breadcrumbs
(regular or gluten-free)

¼ cup grated parmesan
cheese

⅛ tsp salt

Pepper to taste

Butter for greasing the pie dish

2 tbsp olive oil for sautéing

DIRECTIONS

1. Preheat oven to 325–350°F.

2. Sauté chopped onions and garlic in olive oil over medium heat until glassy.

3. Add chopped asparagus and sauté until tender, remove from heat.

4. Whisk eggs together while asparagus is cooling.

5. Add sautéed vegetables, panko crumbs, grated parmesan, salt, and pepper to egg mixture and combine with whisk.

6. Generously grease a glass or ceramic pie dish with butter and pour the mixture into the dish.

7. Bake for about 20 minutes or until firm and beginning to turn golden brown.

8. Cool and serve.

To see this recipe come alive in video and for more healthy lunch ideas, visit our online healthy lunch collection: lunch.justcookforkids.com

VEGGIE BREAKFAST OMELET

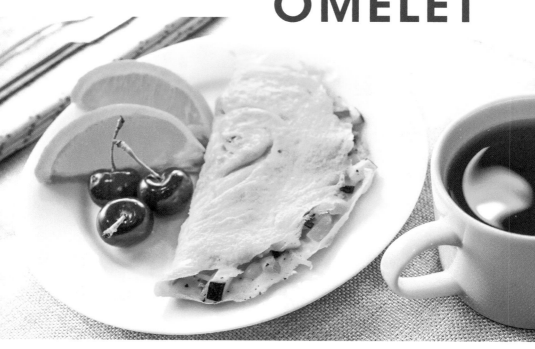

INGREDIENTS

2 eggs

1 small pat of butter

¼ small yellow or white onion, finely chopped

¼ cup grated mozzarella or Monterey Jack cheese

1 cup chopped fresh vegetables of your choice (e.g., baby zucchini, mushrooms, red bell peppers, spinach)

Salt and pepper to taste

DIRECTIONS

1. In a small frying pan, melt half the pat of butter over medium heat. Add the chopped onions and sauté them until they turn glassy, about 2 minutes.

2. While the onions are cooking, whisk the eggs together in a small bowl and set aside.

3. Add the vegetables and sauté them al dente (don't overcook!), about 2 minutes. Remove the vegetables from the pan and set aside.

4. Return the pan to the heat and melt the rest of the butter.

5. Pour the egg mixture into the pan and gently move the cooked portion inward so that all of the egg begins to solidify. Add small amounts of salt and pepper as desired.

6. Layer the cooked vegetables with grated cheese on one half of the omelet.

7. Fold omelet closed and transfer onto a plate.

To see this recipe come alive in video and for more healthy breakfast ideas, visit our online healthy breakfast collection: breakfast.justcookforkids.com

CHICKEN AND YELLOW RICE BALLS

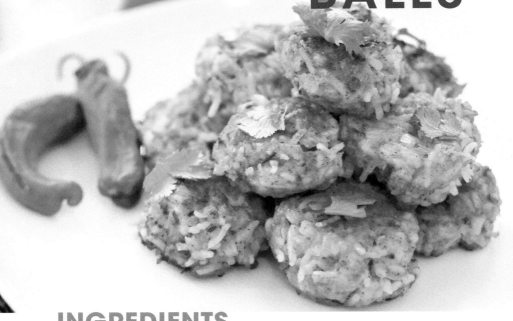

INGREDIENTS

1 lb ground chicken thigh meat

1 tsp mild chili powder

1 tsp salt

2 tsp coriander

1 tsp cumin

¾ tsp turmeric

1 large clove garlic, diced

1 serrano pepper, diced; remove the seeds if you don't want too much heat

¼ yellow onion, finely chopped

1½ cups cooked basmati rice

1 medium sized carrot, shredded

⅓ cup chives, finely chopped

Olive oil for lining the pan

DIRECTIONS

1. Place the ground chicken in a bowl and add mild chili powder, salt, coriander, cumin, turmeric, garlic, serrano, and onions. Mix together the chicken and spices. Add cooked basmati rice, shredded carrots, and fresh chives and mix it all together.

2. Preheat a pan to medium high, with olive oil covering the bottom of the pan.

3. Roll the chicken and rice mixture into little balls about the size of a ping pong ball. Flatten them a little bit to speed up the cooking. Cook the rice balls in the pan and let them sear on the outside for about 5–8 minutes; the seared side should be golden brown. Flip them over on the other side and cook again for 5–8 minutes. Turn the heat down and cook over low heat for 5 more minutes.

4. When the balls are ready, they should be firm to pressure and appear fully cooked on the inside when you cut one open for a testing.

To see this recipe come alive in video and for more healthy dinner ideas, visit our online healthy dinner collection: dinner.justcookforkids.com

SWEET PEA SALAD

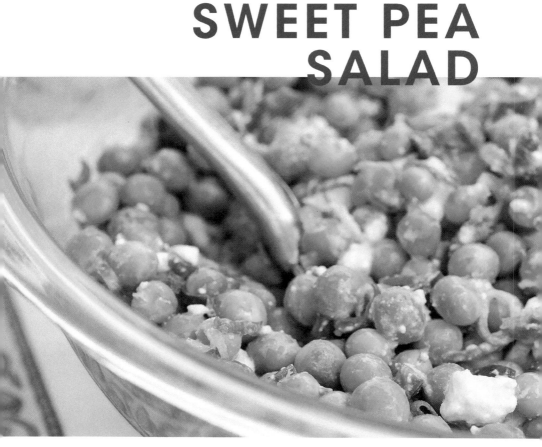

INGREDIENTS

4 cups of fresh shelled English peas (also known as shelling peas or garden peas)

3–4 green onions (scallions), finely chopped

⅓ cup of crumbled sheep's milk feta cheese

2 tbsp of olive oil

1 tsp of fresh lemon juice

¼ cup of finely chopped Kalamata olives

1 pinch of grated lemon rind

Salt and pepper to taste

DIRECTIONS

1. In a saucepan bring approx. 1 inch (2.5 cm) of water to a boil and lower the steamer basket into the pan. While the water is coming to a boil, shell the peas and chop the onions.

2. Allow the peas to steam over boiling water in the steamer basket for approximately 2 minutes.

3. Remove the peas from the steamer and immerse in an ice-water bath to stop the cooking process. Then drain the peas.

4. Transfer the peas into a salad bowl, add the olives, feta cheese, onions, olive oil, lemon juice, lemon rind, and salt and pepper to taste.

5. Toss them all together and enjoy!

To see this recipe come alive in video and for more healthy lunch ideas, visit our online healthy lunch collection: lunch.justcookforkids.com

EGG SALAD SANDWICHES

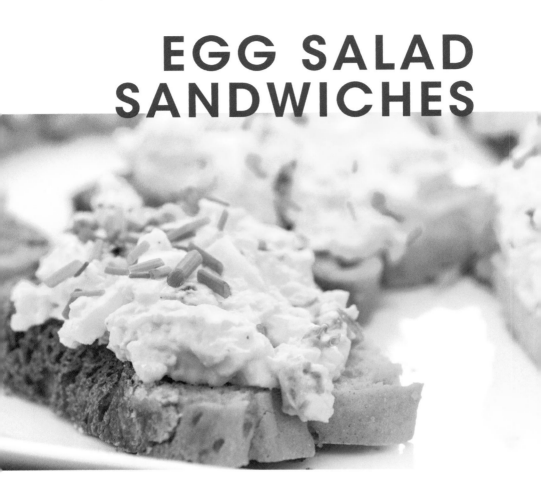

INGREDIENTS

6 eggs

⅓ cup mayonnaise

2–3 gherkin pickles, chopped

1 small shallot or ¼ red onion

½ bunch of chives

Salt and pepper to taste

Bread for serving (I use gluten-free bread because I have a gluten intolerant child, but any type of bread will work)

DIRECTIONS

1. Place eggs in a small pot of cold water on the stove over medium heat.

2. Once the water starts boiling, allow the eggs to boil for about 12–15 minutes.

3. Remove eggs from the water and allow them to cool (can be placed in the fridge).

4. Peel the eggs, place them in a bowl, and mash them into small chunks with a fork.

5. Add mayonnaise, freshly chopped shallots and pickles, and half of the freshly chopped chives. Add salt and pepper to your liking and mix all the ingredients together.

6. Scoop small amounts of the egg mix onto half slices of bread and garnish with a few chopped chives.

To see this recipe come alive in video and for more healthy lunch ideas, visit our online healthy lunch collection: lunch.justcookforkids.com

CINNAMON BREAD PUDDING

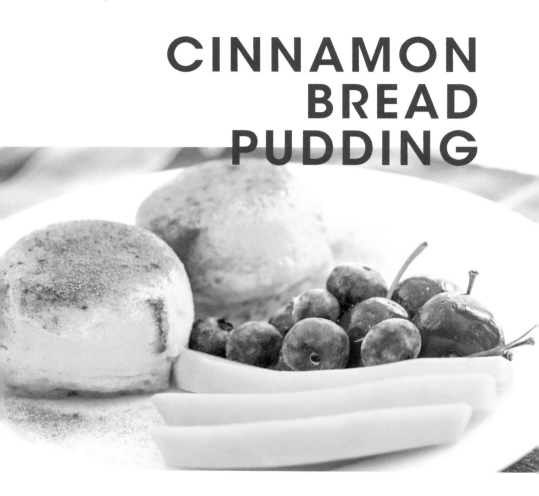

INGREDIENTS

3–4 slices of bread (regular or gluten-free)

unsalted butter

3 eggs

⅓ cup milk

1 tsp vanilla essence (extract)

2 tbsp sugar

2 or 3 shakes of ground cinnamon

Make Sure You Have: A stove-top egg-poacher (a simple covered pot with water at the bottom and six nonstick cups sitting over top to allow steaming will work)

DIRECTIONS

1. Preheat your egg poacher by pouring water in and letting it steam.

2. Cut bread into three thick slices. Butter your bread and cut each slice into quarters.

3. Crack three eggs into a mixing bowl, add in milk, sugar, and vanilla extract. Whisk it together and you have the custard part done.

4. Take a little bit of the butter and place in the egg poacher, and wait until the butter is melted.

5. Take two squares of bread and place them into the cups of the egg-poacher. Fill the cups with the custard mix.

6. Cover and allow the steam to cook the egg for 5 to 7 minutes. In a separate cup, mix cinnamon and sugar to dust on the bread pudding.

7. Once they have risen, use tongs to flip each cup onto a plate, dust them with the cinnamon-sugar mixture, and you're ready to serve!

To see this recipe come alive in video and for more healthy breakfast ideas, visit our online healthy breakfast collection: breakfast.justcookforkids.com

SEA BASS PACKETS

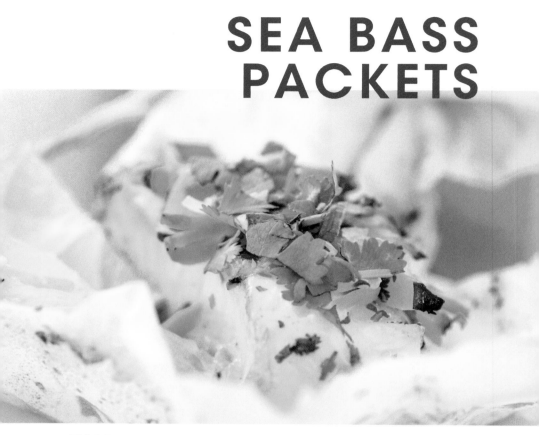

INGREDIENTS

3 lbs Chilean sea bass filets

2 large shallots, chopped finely

2 or 3 large carrots, thinly cut

1 bunch of fresh cilantro, chopped

COOKING SAUCE INGREDIENTS

2 tbsp soy sauce or tamari sauce (gluten-free option)

1 tbsp sesame oil

3 shakes of dried chili flakes

¼ cup lime juice (2 fresh limes)

2 tsp sugar

1 tbsp plum sauce

2 tsp fresh ginger

1 tbsp mirin

Salt and pepper

DIRECTIONS

1. Preheat your oven to 450°F.

Sauce

1. In a medium bowl, mix together lime juice, plum sauce, soy/tamari, sesame oil, sugar, fresh ginger, and mirin.

Sea Bass

1. Chop carrots, shallots, and cilantro.

2. Place a single-serving sized filet of sea bass in the middle of a piece of parchment paper. Sprinkle with a touch of salt and pepper. Drizzle some of the marinade on top of the fish. Sprinkle a tiny bit of the carrots, shallots, and cilantro on top as well.

3. Grab the corners and crunch together to make a bag and tie together with ovenproof string.

4. Make a couple more and place them on a baking sheet and pop them in the oven for 15 minutes.

5. There are two ways to serve. One is to simply cut the string on each package in the kitchen and with a spatula, dish onto a serving plate. Another more theatrical way is to place a package on each plate, bring scissors to the table, and have your guests open up their own goodie bag. Caution—be careful of the steam coming out of the open parchment bag. Add your favorite side, like salad or rice, and serve.

To see this recipe come alive in video and for more healthy dinner ideas, visit our online healthy dinner collection: dinner.justcookforkids.com

GERMAN POTATO SALAD

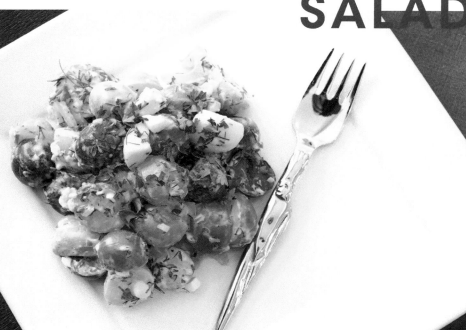

INGREDIENTS

2 lbs small red or Yukon gold potatoes

4 hardboiled eggs

2 tbsp finely chopped fresh parsley

2 tbsp finely chopped fresh dill

1 large shallot, finely chopped or ¼ cup finely chopped red onion

2 stalks of celery, sliced

FOR THE DRESSING

2 tbsp mayonnaise

2 tbsp olive oil

2 tbsp red wine vinegar

1 tbsp Dijon mustard

2 tsp lemon juice

1 tsp salt (more or less as desired)

fresh black pepper (if desired)

DIRECTIONS

1. Boil potatoes for about 10 to 15 minutes in water until a fork can be inserted easily. Cool in refrigerator for 10 to 15 minutes.

2. Boil eggs in water for 7 to 9 minutes. Cool in refrigerator for 10 to 15 minutes.

3. Chop the eggs into quarters or bite-size pieces and cut the potatoes in half and put in a large bowl.

4. Add fresh dill, parsley, celery, and shallots to the bowl, and toss.

5. In a separate bowl, add mayonnaise, mustard, balsamic vinegar, lemon juice, olive oil, and salt and pepper to taste, and mix with a whisk.

6. Pour the dressing over the potato mixture and toss all the ingredients together.

7. Chill well before serving.

To see this recipe come alive in video and for more healthy lunch ideas, visit our online healthy lunch collection: lunch.justcookforkids.com

ALMOND CAKE

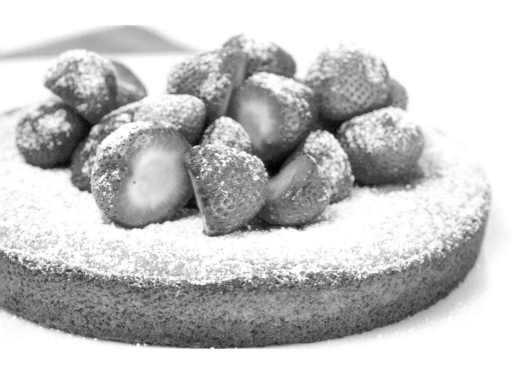

INGREDIENTS

1 stick or 8 tbsp of softened butter

¾ cup sugar

1 tsp vanilla extract

4 eggs

2½ cups almond meal (almond flour)

1½ tsp baking powder

Powdered sugar for dusting (and fresh fruit for decorating if you want)

DIRECTIONS

1. Preheat oven to 325°F.

2. Add the softened butter into the mixer then add sugar and the vanilla extract. Cream together the butter mixture and after couple minutes add in the eggs and blend for a few more minutes.

3. Stop the mixer and add in the almond flour and baking powder. Blend some more.

4. Once the batter is blended well, place it in a cake pan. If you're working with a thick batter, place more in the middle and it will even out in the oven.

5. Flip the cake upside down to take it out of the pan. Place the strawberries on top and dust on some powdered sugar and you're ready to serve!

To see this recipe come alive in video and for more healthy dessert ideas, visit our online healthy dessert collection: dessert.justcookforkids.com

CHOCOLATE STRAWBERRIES

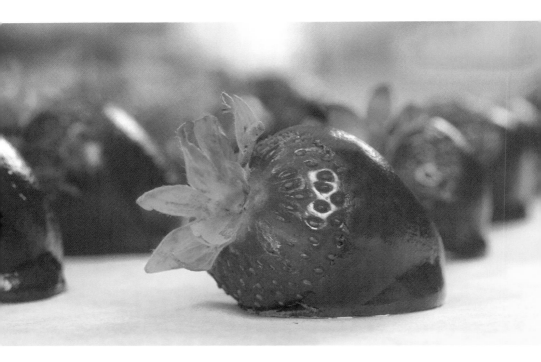

INGREDIENTS

1 packet of good quality semi-sweet chocolate chips

1 box of fresh strawberries

OPTIONAL:

for a softer fondant-style coating, add:

2 tbsp butter and 2 tbsp honey

boiling water

DIRECTIONS

1. Wash and thoroughly dry strawberries.

2. Place chocolate (and optional butter and honey) in a microwave-safe dish and microwave in 30-second intervals (stirring in between). When chocolate is melted, stir the mixture while adding a small amount of boiling water slowly until the texture of the melted chocolate is smooth. For a firmer coating, use only melted chocolate chips for the coating.

3. Hold the strawberries by the stem and dip each one so that they are three-fourths covered by the chocolate mixture. Turn the strawberry for even coating.

4. Lay flat on a piece of parchment paper and allow to cool completely, until outer chocolate coating is firm.

To see this recipe come alive in video and for more healthy dessert ideas, visit our online healthy dessert collection: dessert.justcookforkids.com

REFERENCES

CHAPTER 1

Butte NF. *"Fat Intake of Children in Relation to Energy Requirements."* The American Journal of Clinical Nutrition. *2000;72(5):1246s–1252s.*

Hammons AJ, Fiese BH. *"Is Frequency of Shared Family Meals Related to the Nutritional Health of Children and Adolescents?"* Pediatrics. *2011;127(6):e1565–e1574.*

CHAPTER 2

Kramer, M. and R. Kakuma. *"Optimal Duration of Exclusive Breastfeeding"* (Review). *2007.*

Imdad, A., M.Y. Yakoob, and Z.A. Bhutta. *"Effect of Breastfeeding Promotion Interventions on Breastfeeding Rates, with Special Focus on Developing Countries."* BMC Public Health, *2011. 11(Suppl 3): S24.*

Cope, M.B. and D.B. Allison. *"Critical Review of the World Health Organization's (WHO) 2007 Report on 'Evidence of the Long-term Effects of Breastfeeding: Systematic Reviews and Meta-analysis' with Respect to Obesity."* Obes Rev, *2008. 9(6): 594–605.*

Ip, S., et al. *"Breastfeeding and Maternal and Infant Health Outcomes in Developed Countries."* Evid Rep Technol Assess *(Full Rep), 2007(153): 1–186.*

Apple, R.D. Mothers and Medicine: A Social History of Infant Feeding, 1890–1950. *Vol. 7. 1987: Univ of Wisconsin Press.*

Lanata, C.F., et al. "Global Causes of Diarrheal Disease Mortality in Children <5 Years of Age: A Systematic Review." PLoS One, 2013. 8(9): e72788.

Turin, C.G. and T.J. Ochoa. "The Role of Maternal Breast Milk in Preventing Infantile Diarrhea in the Developing World." Curr Trop Med Rep, 2014. 1(2): 97–105.

Kuhn, L., C. Reitz, and E.J. Abrams. "Breastfeeding and AIDS in the Developing World." Curr Opin Pediatr, 2009. 21(1): 83–93.

CHAPTER 3

Fessler DM, Abrams ET. "Infant Mouthing Behavior: The Immunocalibration Hypothesis." Medical Hypotheses. 2004;63(6):925–932.

Wake M, Hesketh K, Lucas J. "Teething and Tooth Eruption in Infants: A Cohort Study." Pediatrics. 2000;106(6):1374–1379.

Wright CM, Cameron K, Tsiaka M, Parkinson KN. "Is Baby-led Weaning Feasible? When Do Babies First Reach out for and Eat Finger Foods?" Maternal & Child Nutrition. 2011;7(1):27–33.

Picciano MF. "Nutrient Composition of Human Milk." Pediatric Clinics of North America. 2001;48(1):53–67.

Halken S. "Prevention of Allergic Disease in Childhood: Clinical and Epidemiological Aspects of Primary and Secondary Allergy Prevention." Pediatric Allergy and Immunology: Official Publication of the European Society of Pediatric Allergy and Immunology. 2004;15 Suppl 16:4–5, 9–32.

Grimshaw KE, Maskell J, Oliver EM, et al. "Introduction of Complementary Foods and the Relationship to Food Allergy." Pediatrics. 2013;132(6):e1529–1538.

Dovey TM, Staples PA, Gibson EL, Halford JC. "Food Neophobia and 'Picky/Fussy' Eating in Children: A Review." Appetite. 2008;50(2):181–193.

Wardle J, Herrera ML, Cooke L, Gibson EL. "Modifying Children's Food Preferences: The Effects of Exposure and Reward on Acceptance of an Unfamiliar Vegetable." European Journal of Clinical Nutrition. 2003;57(2):341–348.

Mennella JA, Trabulsi JC. "Complementary Foods and Flavor Experiences: Setting the Foundation." Annals of Nutrition & Metabolism. 2012;60 Suppl 2:40–50.

Joneja JM. "Infant Food Allergy Where Are We Now?" Journal of Parenteral and Enteral Nutrition. 2012;36(1 suppl):49S–55S.

Sicherer SH. "Food Allergy." The Lancet. 2002;360(9334):701–710.

"Fish: What Pregnant Women and Parents Should Know." Food and Drug Administration (FDA) and Environmental Protection Agency (EPA). June 2014.

CHAPTER 4

Boeing H, Bechthold A, Bub A, et al. "Critical Review: Vegetables and Fruit in the Prevention of Chronic Diseases." European Journal of Nutrition. 2012;51(6):637–663.

Ledoux T, Hingle M, Baranowski T. "Relationship of Fruit and Vegetable Intake with Adiposity: A Systematic Review." Obesity Reviews. 2011;12(5):e143–e150.

Pearson N, Biddle SJ. "Sedentary Behavior and Dietary Intake in Children, Adolescents, and Adults: A Systematic Review. American Journal of Preventive Medicine. 2011;41(2):178–188.

Evans CE, Christian MS, Cleghorn CL, Greenwood DC, Cade JE. "Systematic Review and Meta-analysis of School-based Interventions to Improve Daily Fruit and Vegetable Intake in Children Aged 5 to 12 y." The American Journal of Clinical Nutrition. 2012;96(4):889–901.

Malik VS, Pan A, Willett WC, Hu FB. "Sugar-sweetened Beverages and Weight Gain in Children and Adults: A Systematic Review and Meta-analysis." The American Journal of Clinical Nutrition. 2013;98(4):1084–1102.

Go A, Mozaffarian D, Roger V. "Sugar-sweetened Beverages Initiatives Can Help Fight Childhood Obesity." Circulation. 2013;127:e6–e245.

Te Morenga L, Mallard S, Mann J. "Dietary Sugars and Body Weight: Systematic Review and Meta-analyses of Randomised Controlled Trials and Cohort Studies." BMJ. 2013;346:e7492.

Xi B, Li S, Liu Z, et al. "Intake of Fruit Juice and Incidence of Type 2 Diabetes: A Systematic Review and Meta-analysis." PloS One. 2014;9(3):e93471.

Sheiham A, James WPT. "A New Understanding of the Relationship Between Sugars, Dental Caries and Fluoride Use: Implications for Limits on Sugars Consumption." Public Health Nutrition. 2014;17(10):2176–2184.

Moynihan P, Kelly S. "Effect on Caries of Restricting Sugars Intake: Systematic Review to Inform WHO Guidelines. Journal of Dental Research. 2013:0022034513508954.

Ludwig DS. "The Glycemic Index: Physiological Mechanisms Relating to Obesity, Diabetes, and Cardiovascular Disease." JAMA: The Journal of the American Medical Association. 2002;287(18):2414–2423.

Hooper L, Summerbell CD, Higgins JP, et al. "Dietary Fat Intake and Prevention of Cardiovascular Disease: Systematic Review." BMJ. 2001;322(7289):757–763.

Moreno JJ, Mitjavila MT. "The Degree of Unsaturation of Dietary Fatty Acids and the Development of Atherosclerosis (Review)." The Journal of Nutritional Biochemistry. 2003;14(4):182–195.

Ornish D, Brown SE, Billings J, et al. "Can Lifestyle Changes Reverse Coronary Heart Disease? The Lifestyle Heart Trial." The Lancet. 1990;336(8708):129–133.

Hu FB, Manson JE, Willett WC. "Types of Dietary Fat and Risk of Coronary Heart Disease: A Critical Review." Journal of the American College of Nutrition. 2001;20(1):5–19.

Oparil S. "Low Sodium Intake—Cardiovascular Health Benefit or Risk?" New England Journal of Medicine. 2014;371(7):677–679.

Dovey TM, Staples PA, Gibson EL, Halford JC. "Food Neophobia and 'Picky/Fussy' Eating in Children: A Review." Appetite. 2008;50(2):181–193.

CHAPTER 5

Cornwell, T.B. and A.R. McAlister. "Alternative Thinking About Starting Points of Obesity: Development of Child Taste Preferences." Appetite, 2011. 56(2): 428–439.

Mustonen, S. and H. Tuorila. "Sensory Education Decreases Food Neophobia Score and Encourages Trying Unfamiliar Foods in 8–12-year-old Children." Food Quality and Preference, 2010. 21(4): 353–360.

Mustonen, S., R. Rantanen, and H. Tuorila. "Effect of Sensory Education on School Children's Food Perception: A 2-year Follow-up Study." Food Quality and Preference, 2009. 20(3): 230–240.

Birch, L., Parker, L., and A. Burns. (Eds.) Early Childhood Obesity Prevention Policies. Committee on Obesity Prevention Policies for Young Children. 2011, Washington, DC: Institute of Medicine of the National Academies, National Academies Press. Dr Leann Lipps Birch is the Distinguished Professor of Human Development and Director of the Center for Childhood Obesity Research at Pennsylvania State University.

A French-language blog on "sensory food education" in Canada: http://mandarine-et-kiwi.blogspot.ca.

Dazeley, P., C. Houston-Price, and C. Hill. "Should Healthy Eating Programmes Incorporate Interaction with Foods in Different Sensory Modalities? A Review of the Evidence." British Journal of Nutrition, 2012. 108(05): 769–777.

Dovey, T.M., et al. "Developmental Differences in Sensory Decision Making Involved in Deciding to Try a Novel Fruit." British Journal of Health Psychology, 2012. 17(2): 258–272.

Kannan, S., et al. "FruitZotic: A Sensory Approach to Introducing Preschoolers to Fresh Exotic Fruits at Head Start Locations in Western Massachusetts." Journal of Nutrition Education and Behavior, 2011. 43(3): 205–206.

Reverdy, C., et al. "Effect of Sensory Education on Willingness to Taste Novel Food in Children." Appetite, 2008. 51(1): 156–165.

Reverdy, C., et al. "Effect of Sensory Education on Food Preferences in Children." Food Quality and Preference, 2010. 21(7): 794–804.

Woo, T. and K.-H. Lee. "Development of a Sensory Education Textbook and Teaching Guidebook for Preference Improvement Toward Traditional Korean Foods in Schoolchildren." Korean Journal of Nutrition, 2011. 44(4): 303–311.

The French Ministry of Education guide is available at: http://alimentation.gouv.fr/IMG/pdf/Classesdugout-formationdesenseignants_cle09fcdb.pdf. For more information on the history of "sensory education" in France, see: http://alimentation.gouv.fr/reseau-education-gout.

CHAPTER 7

For Additional Information

Center for Science in the Public Interest. "Food and Beverage Marketing Survey: Montgomery County Public Schools." http://www.cspinet.org/new/pdf/mcpssurvey.pdf. Accessed October 3, 2014.

Center for Science in the Public Interest. "Nickelodeon: Marketing Obesity to Kids." http://cspinet.org/new/pdf/nickelodeon_brief_2013.pdf. Accessed October 3, 2014.

Center for Science in the Public Interest. "Report Card on Food-marketing Policies: An Analysis of Food and Entertainment Company Policies Regarding Food and Beverage Marketing." http://cspinet.org/new/pdf/marketingreportcard.pdf. Accessed October 16, 2014.

Elliott C. "Assessing 'Fun Foods': Nutritional Content and Analysis of Supermarket Foods Targeted at Children." Obesity Reviews. 2008;9:368–377.

Federal Trade Commission. "A Review of Food Marketing to Children and Adolescents: Follow-up Report." http://www.ftc.gov/sites/default/files/documents/reports/review-food-marketing-children-and-adolescents-follow-report/121221foodmarketingreport.pdf. Accessed October 3, 2014.

Guthrie A. "Mexico Plays the Heavy on Food Ads." The Wall Street Journal. 2014. http://online.wsj.com/articles/mexico-plays-the-heavy-on-junk-food-ads-1408645600. Accessed October 20, 2014.

Healthy Eating Research. "Recommendations for Responsible Food Marketing to Children." http://healthyeatingresearch.org/research/recommendations-for-responsible-food-marketing-to-children/. Accessed May 4, 2015.

John DR. "Consumer Socialization of Children: A Retrospective Look at Twenty-five Years of Research." Journal of Consumer Research. 1999;26:183–213.

Kunkel D, Wilcox BL, Cantor J, Palmer E, Linn S, Dowrick P. "Report of the APA Task Force on Advertising and Children." 2004. http://www.apa.org/pi/families/resources/advertising-children.pdf. Accessed October 3, 2014.

Sorensen H. Inside the Mind of the Shopper: The Science of Retailing. Upper Saddle River, NJ: Wharton School Publishing; 2009.

World Health Organization. "Set of Recommendations on the Marketing of Foods and Non-alcoholic Beverages to Children." http://whqlibdoc.who.int/publications/2010/9789241500210_eng.pdf?ua=1. Accessed October 16, 2014.

CHAPTER 8

Mills C, van Ree R, Breteneder H. "Food Allergy and Intolerance in Europe—Future Directions within the ERA." Allergen Bureau Website. Available at: http://www.allergenbureau.net/downloads/projects-and-resources/Food_Allergy_in_Europe.pdf.

Chafen, J.J.S., et al. "Diagnosing and Managing Common Food Allergies: A Systematic Review." JAMA, 2010. **303**(18): 1848–1856.

"Food Allergy and Food Intolerance." European Food Information Council Website. Available at: http://www.eufic.org/article/en/expid/basics-food-allergy-intolerance/.

Shek, L.P.-C. and B.W. Lee. "Food Allergy in Asia." Current Opinion in Allergy and Clinical Immunology, 2006. **6**(3): 197–201.

De Filippo, C., et al. "Impact of Diet in Shaping Gut Microbiota Revealed by a Comparative Study in Children from Europe and Rural Africa." Proceedings of the National Academy of Sciences, 2010. **107**(33): 14691–14696.

Fishbein, A.B. and R.L. Fuleihan. "The Hygiene Hypothesis Revisited: Does Exposure to Infectious Agents Protect Us from Allergy?" Current Opinion in Pediatrics, 2012. **24**(1): 98–102.

Du Toit, G., et al. "Early Consumption of Peanuts in Infancy Is Associated with a Low Prevalence of Peanut Allergy." Journal of Allergy and Clinical Immunology, 2008. **122**(5): 984–991.

Wang, J.-Y., et al. "Acetaminophen and/or Antibiotic Use in Early Life and the Development of Childhood Allergic Diseases." International Journal of Epidemiology, 2013. **42**(4): 1087–1099.

Hong, X., et al. "Genome-wide Association Study Identifies Peanut Allergy-specific Loci and Evidence of Epigenetic Mediation in US Children." Nature Communications, 2015. **6**.

Greer, F.R., S.H. Sicherer, and A.W. Burks. "Effects of Early Nutritional Interventions on the Development of Atopic Disease in Infants and Children: The Role of Maternal Dietary Restriction, Breastfeeding, Timing of Introduction of Complementary Foods, and Hydrolyzed Formulas." Pediatrics, 2008. **121**(1): 183–191.

Friedman, N.J. and R.S. Zeiger. "The Role of Breast-feeding in the Development of Allergies and Asthma." Journal of Allergy and Clinical Immunology, 2005. **115**(6): 1238–1248.

Nadeau, K.C., et al. "Oral Immunotherapy and Anti-IgE Antibody-adjunctive Treatment for Food Allergy." Immunology and Allergy Clinics of North America, 2012. **32**(1): 111–133.

CHAPTER 9

De Onis, M., M. Blössner, and E. Borghi. "Global Prevalence and Trends of Overweight and Obesity Among Preschool Children." The American Journal of Clinical Nutrition, 2010. **92**(5): 1257–1264.

"Obesity Update," L.a.S.A. OECD Directorate for Employment, Editor. 2014.

Singh, A.S. et al. "Tracking of Childhood Overweight into Adulthood: A Systematic Review of the Literature." Obesity Reviews, 2008. **9**(5): 474–488.

Walls, H.L. et al. "Obesity and Trends in Life Expectancy." Journal of Obesity, 2012. **2012**.

Holtcamp, W. "Obesogens: An Environmental Link to Obesity." Environ Health Perspect, 2012. **120**(2):a62–a68.

"Basics About Childhood Obesity." 2012, US Centers for Disease Control.

Bassali, R. et al. "Utility of Waist Circumference Percentile for Risk Evaluation in Obese Children." International Journal of Pediatric Obesity, 2010. **5**(1): 97–101.

Janssen, I., P.T. Katzmarzyk, and R. Ross. "Waist Circumference and Not Body Mass Index Explains Obesity-related Health Risk." The American Journal of Clinical Nutrition, 2004. **79**(3): 379–384.

Barlow, S.E. "Expert Committee Recommendations Regarding the Prevention, Assessment, and Treatment of Child and Adolescent Overweight and Obesity: Summary Report." Pediatrics, 2007. **120**(Supplement 4): S164–S192.

"What Is Metabolic Syndrome?" NIH: National Heart, Lung, and Blood Institute. Available from http://www.nhlbi.nih.gov/health/health-topics/topics/ms/.

Messiah, S. et al. "The Imperative to Prevent and Treat Childhood Obesity: Why the World Cannot Afford to Wait." Clinical Obesity, 2013. **3**(6): 163–171.

Riley, M.R. et al. "Underdiagnosis of Pediatric Obesity and Underscreening for Fatty Liver Disease and Metabolic Syndrome by Pediatricians and Pediatric Subspecialists." The Journal of Pediatrics, 2005. 147(6): 839–842.

Spear BA, B.S., Ervin C, Ludwig DS, Saelens BE, Schetzina KE, Taveras EM. "Recommendations for Treatment of Child and Adolescent Overweight and Obesity." Pediatrics, 2007. **120**(Supplemental 4): S254–88.

Stallings, V.a.U., R. "Gut, Fat, Iron, and Brain: Where Are We?" Satellite Symposium of the 2008 World Congress of Pediatric Gastroenterology, Hepatology, and Nutrition August 17, 2008, Iguassu, Brazil. Journal of Pediatric Gastroenterology and Nutrition, 2009. **48**(S1).

Arenz, S. et al. "Breast-feeding and Childhood Obesity: A Systematic Review." International Journal of Obesity, 2004. **28**(10): 1247–1256.

Sonneville, K.R. et al. "Juice and Water Intake in Infancy and Later Beverage Intake and Adiposity: Could Juice Be a Gateway Drink?" Obesity, 2015. **23**(1): 170–176.

Yang, Q. "Gain Weight by 'Going Diet?' Artificial Sweeteners and the Neurobiology of Sugar Cravings: Neuroscience 2010." The Yale Journal of Biology and Medicine, 2010. **83**(2): 101.

Lenoir, M. et al. "Intense Sweetness Surpasses Cocaine Reward." PloS One, 2007. **2**(8): e698.

Redman, L.M. et al. "Metabolic and Behavioral Compensations in Response to Caloric Restriction: Implications for the Maintenance of Weight Loss." PloS One, 2009. **4**(2): e4377.

Guyenet, S.J. and M.W. Schwartz. "Regulation of Food Intake, Energy Balance, and Body Fat Mass: Implications for the Pathogenesis and Treatment of Obesity." The Journal of Clinical Endocrinology & Metabolism, 2012. **97**(3): 745–755.

Durrant, M.L. et al. "Factors Influencing the Composition of the Weight Lost by Obese Patients on a Reducing Diet." British Journal of Nutrition, 1980. **44**(03): 275–285.

Kroeger, C.M., K.K. Hoddy, and K.A. Varady. "Impact of Weight Regain on Metabolic Disease Risk: A Review of Human Trials." Journal of Obesity, 2014. **2014**.

Van Ittersum, K. and B. Wansink. "Plate Size and Color Suggestibility: The Delboeuf Illusion's Bias on Serving and Eating Behavior." Journal of Consumer Research, 2012. **39**(2): 215–228.

Almiron-Roig, E. et al. "Estimating Food Portions: Influence of Unit Number, Meal Type and Energy Density." Appetite, 2013. **71**: 95–103.

Mitchell, J.A. et al. "Greater Screen Time Is Associated with Adolescent Obesity: A Longitudinal Study of the BMI Distribution from Ages 14 to 18. Obesity, 2013. **21**(3): 572–575.

American Academy of Pediatrics. "Policy Statement: Children, Adolescents, Obesity, and the Media." Pediatrics, 2011. **128**(1): 201–208.

Quattrin, T. et al. "Treatment Outcomes of Overweight Children and Parents in the Medical Home." Pediatrics, 2014. **134**(2): 290–297.

Cooke, L. "The Importance of Exposure for Healthy Eating in Childhood: A Review." Journal of Human Nutrition and Dietetics, 2007. **20**(4): 294–301.

van der Horst, K., A. Ferrage, and A. Rytz. "Involving Children in Meal Preparation: Effects on Food Intake." Appetite, 2014. **79**: 18–24.

Cespedes, E.M. et al. "Longitudinal Associations of Sleep Curtailment with Metabolic Risk in Mid-childhood." Obesity, 2014. **22**(12): 2586–2592.

Donga, E. et al. "A Single Night of Partial Sleep Deprivation Induces Insulin Resistance in Multiple Metabolic Pathways in Healthy Subjects." The Journal of Clinical Endocrinology & Metabolism, 2010. **95**(6): 2963–2968.

Reilly, J.J. et al. "Early Life Risk Factors for Obesity in Childhood: Cohort Study." BMJ, 2005. **330**(7504): 1357.

Landhuis, C.E. et al. "Childhood Sleep Time and Long-term Risk for Obesity: A 32-year Prospective Birth Cohort Study." Pediatrics, 2008. **122**(5): 955–960.

"Children and Sleep." National Sleep Foundation, Available from: http://sleepfoundation.org/sleep-topics/children-and-sleep/page/0/2.

Pellis, S.M. and V.C. Pellis. "Rough-and-tumble Play and the Development of the Social Brain." Current Directions in Psychological Science, *2007.* **16***(2): 95–98.*

CHAPTER 10

(USDA), U.S.D.o.A., National Count of Farmers Market Directory Listings. 2014.

Canning, P. "A Revised and Expanded Food Dollar Series: A Better Understanding of Our Food Costs," U.S.D.o.A.E.R. Service, Editor. 2011.

Agency, U.E.P. "Overview of Greenhouse Gases: Nitrous Oxide Emissions." Available from http://epa.gov/climatechange/ghgemissions/gases/n2o.html.

Diaz, R.J. and R. Rosenberg. "Spreading Dead Zones and Consequences for Marine Ecosystems." Science, *2008.* **321***(5891): 926–929.*

Arcury, T.A., S.A. Quandt, and A. Dearry. "Farmworker Pesticide Exposure and Community-based Participatory Research: Rationale and Practical Applications." Environmental Health Perspectives, *2001.* **109** *(Suppl 3): 429.*

McCauley, L.A. et al. "Studying Health Outcomes in Farmworker Populations Exposed to Pesticides." Environmental Health Perspectives, *2006:953–960.*

Bouchard, M.F. et al. "Prenatal Exposure to Organophosphate Pesticides and IQ in 7-year-old Children." Environmental Health Perspectives, *2011.*

Engel, S.M. et al. "Prenatal Exposure to Organophosphates, Paraoxonase 1, and Cognitive Development in Childhood." Environmental Health Perspectives, *2011.*

Rauh, V. et al. "Seven-year Neurodevelopmental Scores and Prenatal Exposure to Chlorpyrifos, a Common Agricultural Pesticide." Environmental Health Perspectives, *2011.* **119***(8): 1196.*

Miranda, J. et al. "Antimicrobial Resistance in Enterobacteriaceae Strains Isolated from Organic Chicken, Conventional Chicken and Conventional Turkey Meat: A Comparative Survey." Food Control, *2008.* **19***(4): 412–416.*

"Living Planet Report 2010: Biodiversity, Biocapacity, and Development." D. Pollard, Editor. 2010, World Wildlife Fund, Global Footprint Network, Zoological Society of London.

Janzen, D.H. "Dispersal of Small Seeds by Big Herbivores: Foliage Is the Fruit." American Naturalist, *1984: 338–353.*

Pollan, M. "Power steer." New York Times Magazine, 2002. **31.**

"Tackling Climate Change Through Livestock: A Global Assessment of Emissions and Mitigation Opportunities." 2013, Food and Agriculture Organization of the United Nations.

Schardt, D. "Going Organic, in Nutrition Action Healthletter." 2012, Center for Science in the Public Interest: Washington, DC. 3–8.

Mellon M, B.C., Benbrook KL. "Hogging It: Estimates of Antimicrobial Abuse in Livestock." 2001, Union of Concerned Scientists.

Mekonnen, M.M. and A.Y. Hoekstra. "A Global Assessment of the Water Footprint of Farm Animal Products." Ecosystems, *2012. 15(3): 401–415.*

Mekonnen MM, H.A. "The Green, Blue and Grey Water Footprint of Farm Animals and Animal Products: Value of Water Research Report," in Value of Water Research Report Series. 2010, UNESCO-IHE Institute for Water Education: Netherlands.

Hoekstra, A.Y. "The Hidden Water Resource Use Behind Meat and Dairy." Animal Frontiers, 2012. **2**(2): 3–8.

Mozaffarian, D. and E.B. Rimm. "Fish Intake, Contaminants, and Human Health: Evaluating the Risks and the Benefits." JAMA, 2006. **296**(15): 1885–1899.

Torpy, J.M., C. Lynm, and R.M. Glass. "Eating Fish: Health Benefits and Risks." JAMA, 2006. **296**(15): 1926–1926.

Myers, R.A. and B. Worm. "Extinction, Survival or Recovery of Large Predatory Fishes." Philosophical Transactions of the Royal Society B: Biological Sciences, 2005. **360**(1453): 13–20.

"Fish: Friend or Foe." Harvard School of Public Health. Available from http://www.hsph.harvard.edu/nutritionsource/fish/.

"Seafood & Your Health. Monterey Bay Aquarium Seafood Watch." Available from http://www.seafood-watch.org/consumers/seafood-and-your-health.

Ottolenghi, F. "Capture-based Aquaculture of Bluefin Tuna." Global Overview. FAO Fisheries Technical Paper, 2008. **508**: 169–182.

"What Is the Meaning of 'Natural' on the Label of Food?" US Food and Drug Administration. 2015; Available from http://www.fda.gov/aboutfda/transparency/basics/ucm214868.htm.

Cynthia, D. et al. "A Review of Fatty Acid Profiles and Antioxidant Content in Grass-fed and Grain-fed Beef." Nutrition Journal, 2010.

CHAPTER 11

Ventura, A.K. and J. Worobey. "Early Influences on the Development of Food Preferences." Current Biology, 2013. **23**(9): R401–R408.

Beauchamp, G.K. and J.A. Mennella. "Flavor Perception in Human Infants: Development and Functional Significance." Digestion, 2011. **83**(Suppl 1): 1.

Cooke, L. and A. Fildes. "The Impact of Flavour Exposure In Utero and During Milk Feeding on Food Acceptance at Weaning and Beyond." Appetite, 2011. **57**(3): 808–811.

http://www.choosemyplate.gov/pregnancy-breastfeeding/pregnancy-nutritional-needs.html

Sokol, R.J., V. Delaney-Black, and B. Nordstrom. "Fetal Alcohol Spectrum Disorder." JAMA, 2003. **290**(22): 2996–2999.

Henderson, J., U. Kesmodel, and R. Gray. "Systematic Review of the Fetal Effects of Prenatal Binge-drinking." Journal of Epidemiology and Community Health, 2007. **61**(12): 1069–1073.

Barr, H.M. et al. "Binge Drinking During Pregnancy as a Predictor of Psychiatric Disorders on the Structured Clinical Interview for DSM-IV in Young Adult Offspring." The American Journal of Psychiatry, 2006. **163**(6): 1061–1065.

Little, R.E. "Moderate Alcohol Use During Pregnancy and Decreased Infant Birth Weight." American Journal of Public Health, 1977. **67**(12): 1154–1156.

Hanson, J.W., A.P. Streissguth, and D.W. Smith. "The Effects of Moderate Alcohol Consumption During Pregnancy on Fetal Growth and Morphogenesis." Journal of Pediatrics, 1978. **92**(3): 457–460.

Little, R.E. and J.K. Wendt. "The Effects of Maternal Drinking in the Reproductive Period: An Epidemiologic Review." Journal of Substance Abuse, 1991. **3**(2): 187–204.

Lazzaroni, F. et al. "Moderate Maternal Drinking and Outcome of Pregnancy." European Journal of Epidemiology, 1993. **9**(6): 599–606.

Lundsberg, L.S., M.B. Bracken, and A.F. Saftlas. "Low-to-moderate Gestational Alcohol Use and Intrauterine Growth Retardation, Low Birthweight, and Preterm Delivery." Annals of Epidemiology, 1997. **7**(7): 498–508.

Bowen, D.J. "Taste and Food Preference Changes Across the Course of Pregnancy." Appetite, 1992. **19**(3): 233–242.

Myaruhucha, C. "Food Cravings, Aversions and Pica Among Pregnant Women in Dar es Salaam, Tanzania." Tanzania Journal of Health Research, 2009. **11**(1).

Hook, E.B. "Dietary Cravings and Aversions During Pregnancy." The American Journal of Clinical Nutrition, 1978. **31**(8): 1355–1362.

Fekete, K. et al. "Effect of Folate Intake on Health Outcomes in Pregnancy: A Systematic Review and Meta-analysis on Birth Weight, Placental Weight and Length of Gestation." Nutr J, 2012. **11**(1): 75.

Haider, B.A. et al. "Anaemia, Prenatal Iron Use, and Risk of Adverse Pregnancy Outcomes: Systematic Review and Meta-analysis." BMJ, 2013. **346**.

Abbaspour, N., R. Hurrell, and R. Kelishadi. "Review on Iron and Its Importance for Human Health." Journal of Research in Medical Sciences: The Official Journal of Isfahan University of Medical Sciences, 2014. **19**(2): 164.

Larqué, E. et al. "Omega 3 Fatty Acids, Gestation and Pregnancy Outcomes." British Journal of Nutrition, 2012. **107**(S2): S77–S84.

Olmedo, P. et al. "Determination of Toxic Elements (Mercury, Cadmium, Lead, Tin and Arsenic) in Fish and Shellfish Samples: Risk Assessment for the Consumers." Environment International, 2013. **59**: 63–72.

Zimmermann, M. and F. Delange. "Iodine Supplementation of Pregnant Women in Europe: A Review and Recommendations." European Journal of Clinical Nutrition, 2004. **58**(7): 979–984.

Zimmermann, M.B. "Iodine Deficiency in Pregnancy and the Effects of Maternal Iodine Supplementation on the Offspring: A Review." The American Journal of Clinical Nutrition, 2009. **89**(2): 668S–672S.

Organization, W.H. "Assessment of Iodine Deficiency Disorders and Monitoring Their Elimination: A Guide for Programme Managers." 2007.

Specker, B. "Vitamin D Requirements During Pregnancy." The American Journal of Clinical Nutrition, 2004. **80**(6): 1740S–1747S.

Yaktine, A.L. and K.M. Rasmussen. "Weight Gain During Pregnancy: Reexamining the Guidelines." 2009: National Academies Press.

Sridhar, S.B. et al. "Maternal Gestational Weight Gain and Offspring Risk for Childhood Overweight or Obesity." American Journal of Obstetrics and Gynecology, 2014. **211**(3): 259. e1–259. e8.

http://www.eatright.org/resource/health/pregnancy/prenatal-wellness/healthy-weight-during-pregnancy

CREDITS

CHAPTER 1

CHAPTER 2

CHAPTER 3

3.1 Copyright in the Public Domain.
3.2 Copyright in the Public Domain.
3.3 Copyright in the Public Domain.
3.4 Copyright © tigerpuppala (CC by 2.0) at http://commons.wikimedia.org/wiki/File%3AFirst_rice.jpg.
3.5 Copyright in the Public Domain.

CHAPTER 4

4.1 Centers for Disease Control and Prevention, U.S. Department of Health & Human Services, "Growth Chart," WHO Child Growth Standards. Copyright in the Public Domain.
4.2 Copyright in the Public Domain.
4.3 Copyright in the Public Domain.
4.4 Copyright in the Public Domain.
4.5 Copyright in the Public Domain.
4.6.1 Copyright in the Public Domain.
4.6.2 Copyright in the Public Domain.
4.6.3 Copyright in the Public Domain.

CHAPTER 5

5.1 Copyright © Depositphotos/monkeybusiness.
5.3a Copyright © Depositphotos/matka_Wariatka.
5.3b Copyright © Depositphotos/matka_Wariatka.

CHAPTER 7

7.1 Copyright in the Public Domain.
7.2.1 Copyright in the Public Domain.
7.2.2 Copyright in the Public Domain.
7.2.3 Copyright in the Public Domain.
7.3 Copyright in the Public Domain.
7.5 Aviva Musicus, Aner Tal, and Brian Wansink, Food and Brand Lab, Cornell University, "Eyes in the Aisles: Why is Cap'n Crunch Looking Down at My Child?" Environment & Behavior, (2014). URL: http://foodpsychology.cornell.edu/op/cerealeyes. Copyright © 2014 by Food and Brand Lab, Cornell University. Reprinted with permission.
7.6 Copyright © Mamoritai (CC BY-SA 2.0) at https://www.flickr.com/photos/mamoritai/3437088496/.
7.7 U.S. Department of Agriculture, "Smart Snacks in School," http://www.fns.usda.gov/sites/default/files/allfoods_infographic.pdf. Copyright in the Public Domain.

CHAPTER 11

CPSIA information can be obtained at www.ICGtesting.com
Printed in the USA
LVIW01n0319211015
459066LV00001B/1